RATIONAL FASTING

for PHYSICAL, MENTAL &
SPIRITUAL REJUVENATION

By
Prof. Arnold Ehret

Published by
EHRET LITERATURE PUBLISHING CO., INC.
Dobbs Ferry, NY 10522-0024

Fifteenth Edition
Copyright © 1926, 1938, 1966, 1987, 1994
EHRET LITERATURE PUBLISHING CO., INC.
Dobbs Ferry, NY 10522-0024
Printed in U.S.A.

This book is an AUTHENTIC copy of the ORIGINAL version of Professor Arnold Ehret's RATIONAL FASTING FOR PHYSICAL, MENTAL AND SPIRITUAL REJUVENATION. For information about other Ehret publications, the Ehret Health Club or newsletter write to:

EHRET LITERATURE PUBLISHING CO., INC.
P.O. Box 24
Dobbs Ferry, NY 10522-0024

RATIONAL FASTING

Sections II and III were originally published in booklet form under the titles ROADS TO HEALTH AND HAPPINESS and THE DEFINITE CURE OF CHRONIC CONSTIPATION.

Introduction

Theories of life abound, but the immutable laws by which humans, all organisms, and the universe function have not changed over the past century, nor the millennia. If you desire true health and inner contentment seek out what actually works, and indeed, what has always worked.

In this classic and inspirational book, Prof. Arnold Ehret reminds us of our innate ability to heal any ailment, and live the "Paradise Health" that is each of our birthright. He states clearly and simply the basic tenets by which all living beings lead vibrant, pain-free, disease-free lives, yet humans seem to have forgotten.

RATIONAL FASTING and its companion THE MUSCUSLESS DIET HEALING SYSTEM have inspired millions, since their first publication in the 1910's, to live a life brimming with health. They are the catalysts that inspired many prominent people in today's raw foods revolution such as Joe Alexander, Gabriel Cousens, M.D., Dick Gregory, Aris Latham, Steve Meyerowitz, David Wolfe, and more.

To fast correctly and form dietary and lifestyle habits which bring truly robust health, one must gain the proper knowledge and have the courage to carry it forth. Ehret provides us with both. In the present *misinformation age*, where disease consciousness and nutritional confusion are the norm, his convictions are more needed than ever.

How many fasters have lived with this book close at hand, highlighted its words, dog-eared its pages, and felt Ehret's passion for a vital life? How many have understood Ehret's desire that the highest levels of health which he attained, could and should be attained by all?

One of Prof. Ehret's oft repeated maxims was, "whatever simple reason cannot grasp is humbug, however scientific it may sound." Can sense be made of today's interminable wash of health advice— new surgery, miracle drug, alternative therapy, co-enzyme, neutraceutical, high-protein diet, etc. The medical science and alternative health practices spew an endless litany of theories and techniques oblivious to, or barely aware of, the unchanging laws of health. The results have been at best short-term alleviation of symptoms, and at worst detrimental and deadly.

When making decisions, look at what actually works. Rather than accepting the hype and feeling stunned by today's media-daze, find out what results people are in fact getting. If they are not receiving the results you want, don't listen to them. And certainly don't do what they say!

Evidence the "War On Cancer." Since this campaign began in

1971, despite loudly heralded medical advances, annual cancer deaths in America have more than doubled to one out of three today. Regarding the typical treatment, how often has it been said, "The cure is worse than the disease." Over 100 billion dollars is wasted each year, and the "War" has proven to be a cruel hoax pulling at the heartstrings and emptying the pockets of sufferers and their families alike.

In contrast, many have cured themselves of this scourge by fasting and closely following a raw vegan diet (no animals or animal-products) or living foods diet; modern terms for Ehret's mucusless diet. The same is true of every disease, and Prof. Ehret explains plainly and concisely why.

This book is about attaining full "Paradise Health." It is not about "moderation." If you want a moderate amount of health, then follow its directions moderately. But if you desire a buoyant and glowingly vital life, follow its directions to the full. All people, no matter what their age and situation, can and should have this. When it comes to health, there is no valor in compromise.

RATIONAL FASTING is the light which for me illumined the path to deep-seeded well-being. It brought me clearly to the realizations that cooked and processed foods are poisons; that the only real foods for humans are fresh, uncooked fruits and vegetables; that fasting is the law of cure by which all in the community of life heal; and that true health can only be achieved by one's own energies and actions. I am so humbly thankful because today I enjoy a level of robust health undreamed of in my earlier life. This is the experience of so many in the burgeoning raw foods movement, for whom Ehret continues to be an inspirational beacon.

If you understand Prof. Arnold Ehret's simple and truthful message, then take action and live it. Take the knowledge, be wise in your decisions, remain undeterred by the naysayers (who will often be those closest to you), be inspired, and achieve your "Paradise Health." With a little effort you will find many to support you along the way. Today there are raw food restaurants, raw food retreats, fasting centers, growers of high-quality organic fruits and vegetables, uncook books, raw food pot luck dinners, and raw food support groups across the world. Just be sure they are following the tenets herein.

There is no single greater contribution you can make to your health and the well-being of the Earth than to fast and live a raw vegan diet. It is the quiet revolution, and slowly and steadily it is happening.

Enjoy this book! I hope it will inspire you, as it has me, to create the physically, mentally, and spiritually vibrant life we all deserve.

Robert A. Miller
March 6, 2000

Preface

Are you one of the thousands of present age persons—discouraged and disheartened because of ill-health; is your faith in so-called cures shattered after having tried them without results; are you only able to use a small percent of the vitality that good Mother Nature endows her beloved ones with? Probably you have been told that only an operation will save you. Somehow, when we suffer organic trouble we fail to think clearly and permit ourselves to be easily persuaded into operations. If you are one of these unfortunates DON'T GIVE UP HOPE. For "he that hath health hath hope, and he that hath hope, hath everything."

"Since man degenerated through civilization, he no longer knows what to do when he becomes sick". The genuine principles of healing are simple and few. Our very lack of appetite which occurs when we are sick is Nature's method of teaching her children. One might properly call this a "forced fast". These are but a few of the truisms taught by Arnold Ehret in his many writings. Our greatest possession is health.

A general agreement seems to be gaining acceptance among an increasing number of Practitioners both of the drugless as well as the medical fraternity that the fundamental cause of disease is the presence of foreign material in the human body, but it has not as yet led to the discovery of the roots of this invading mystery. Prof. Ehret has conclusively proven that this disease causing material is the undigested, uneliminated and decayed, rotting food elements resulting from too much eating of wrong foods. It is therefore entirely reasonable and should be clearly seen that the main factor in the health enigma should consist of dietetics. If over-eating is the main cause of the patient's disease, it requires intelligently conducted fast's to correct the condition. It is a known fact that all of the animal kingdom living in a natural environment, instinctively heal themselves through fasting. It can be easily proven that persons living on a mixed diet of animal flesh and starchy vegetables, has a system more of less clogged with mucus. This condition has been going on since early childhood, — in fact even before. These foods are not suitable for mankind, and they form a sticky, gluey consistency which eventually clogs the circulation. Is it not self-evident and certainly reasonable that this disease-producing eating must be stopped! Fasting, plus a decrease in the quantity of food eaten daily is the only check on over-eating. Exercise due precaution not to proceed too rapidly for an unwise application of the eliminative process could cause a serious condition to develope.

This drugless healing is not limited in its scope; and thru its proper application and use it restores normal functioning overcoming practically all ailments to which the human-family is subject.

"TRUTH WEARS NO MASK; BOWS AT NO HUMAN SHRINE: SEEKS NEITHER PLACE NOR APPLAUSE: SHE ASKS ONLY A HEARING." — Redfield.

Contents

Frontispiece, ARNOLD EHRET

Part I

Part II

Part III

The Common Fundamental Cause in the Nature of Diseases

BY PROF. ARNOLD EHRET

All the phases of the process of development of the medical science including those of the earliest periods of civilization, have in their way of understanding the causal nature of diseases, that one thing in common i.e.: that the diseases, owing to external causes, enter into the human body and thus, by force of a necessary or at least unavoidable law, disturb the body in its existence, cause it pain and at last destroy it. Even modern medical science, no matter how scientifically enlightened it pretends to be, has not quite turned away from this basic note of demoniac interpretation. In fact, the most modern achievement, bacteriology, rejoices over every newly discovered bacillus as a further addition to the army of beings whose accepted task it is to endanger the life of man.

Looking at it from a philosophical standpoint, this interpretation differs from the mediaeval superstition and the period of fetishism only in the supplemental name. Formerly it was an "evil spirit," which imagination went so far as to believe in "satanic personages"; now this same dangerous monster is a microscopically visible being whose existence has been proven beyond any doubt.

The matter, it is true, has still a great drawback in the so-called "disposition" — a fine word! — But what we really are to understand by it, nobody has ever told us. All the tests on animals, with their symptom-reactions, do not prove anything sure, because these occur only by means of injection into the blood-circulation and never by introduction into the digestive channel through the mouth.

There is something true in the conception of "external invasion" of a disease, as well as in heredity, however not in the sense that the invader is a spirit (demon) hostile to life, or a microscopic being (bacillus); but all *diseases* without exception, even the hereditary, are caused — disregarding a few other hygienic causes — by biologically wrong, "unnatural" food and by each ounce of over-nourishment, only and exclusively.

First of all I maintain that in all diseases without exception there exists a tendency by the organism to secrete mucus, and in case of a more advanced stage — pus (decomposed blood). Of course every healthy organism must also contain a certain mucus — lymph, a fatty substance of the bowels, etc., of a mucus nature. Every expert will admit this in all catarrhalic cases, from a harmless cold in the nose to inflammation of the lungs and consumption, as well as in epilepsy (attacks showing froth at the mouth, mucus). Where this secretion of mucus does not show freely and openly, as in cases of ear, eye, skin or stomach trouble, heart diseases, rheumatism, gout, etc., even in all degrees of insanity, mucus is the main factor of the illness. The natural secretive-organs unable to cope with it longer, the mucus enters the blood causing heat, inflammation, pain and fever at the respective spot where the vessel-system is probably contracted owing to an over-cooling fever (cold), heat, inflammation, pain, fever, etc.

We need only to give a patient of any kind nothing but "mucusless" food, for instance; fruit or even nothing but water or lemonade; we then find that the entire digestive energy, freed for the first time, throws itself upon the mucus-matters, accumulated since childhood and frequently hardened, as well as on the "pathologic beds" formed therefrom. And the result? With unconditional certainty this mucus which I mark as the common basic and main cause of all diseases will appear in the urine and in the excrements. If the disease is already somewhat advanced so that in some spot, even in the innermost interior, there have appeared pathologic beds, i.e., decomposed cellular tissues, then pus is also being secreted. As soon as the introduction of mucus by means of "artificial food," fat meat, bread, potatoes, farinaceous products, rice, milk, etc., ceases, the blood-circulation attacks the mucus and the pus of the body themselves and secretes them through the urine, and in the case of heavily infected bodies, even through all the openings at their command as well as through the mucus membranes.

If potatoes, grain-meal, rice or the respective meat-materials are boiled long enough, we receive jelly-like slime (mucus) or paste used by bookbinders and carpenters. This mucus substance soon becomes sour, ferments, and forms a bed for fungi, moulds and bacilli. In the process of digestion, which is nothing else but a boiling, a combustion; this slime or paste is being secreted in the same manner, for the blood can use only the exdigested sugar transformed from starch. The secreted matter, the superfluous product, i.e., this paste or slime is being completely excreted in the beginning. It is, therefore, easy to understand that in the course of life the intestines and the stomach are gradually being pasted and slimed up to such an extent that this paste of floral and this slime of faunal origin turn into fermentation, clog up the blood-vessels and finally decompose the stagnated blood. If figs, dates or grapes are boiled down thick enough we also receive a pap which, however, does not turn to fermentation and never secretes slime, but which is called syrup. Fruit-sugar, the most important thing for the blood, is also sticky, it is true, but is being completely used up by the body as the highest form of fuel, and leaves for excretion only traces of cellulose, which, not being sticky, is promptly excreted and does not ferment. Boiled-down sugar, owing to its resistance against fermentation, is even used for the preservation of food.

Each healthy or sick person deposits on the tongue a sticky mucus as soon as he reduces his food or fasts. This occurs also on the mucus membrane of the stomach, of which the tongue is an exact copy. In the first stool after fasting this mucus makes its appearance.

I recommend to my reader or to the physicians and searchers to test my claims by way of experiments which alone are entitled to real scientific recognition. The experiment, the question put to nature, is the basis of a natural science and reveals the infallible truth, no matter whether it is stated by me or somebody else. Furthermore, I recommend the following experiments to those who are brave enough to test on their own bodies which I undertook on mine. They will receive the same answer from nature, i.e., from their organism, provided that the latter be sound in my sense. "Exact" to a certain degree reacts only to the clean, sound, mucusless organism. After a two years' strict fruit-diet with intercalated fasting cures, I had attained a degree of health which is simply not imaginable nowadays and which allowed of my making the following experiments:

With a knife I made an incision in my lower arm; there was no flow of blood as it thickened instantly; closing up the wound, no inflammation, no pain, no mucus and pus:

healed up in three days, blood crust thrown off. Later, with vegetaric food, including mucus-ferments (starch food), but without eggs and milk: The wound bled a little, caused some pain and pussed slightly, a light inflammation, complete healing only after some time. After that the same wounding, with meat-food and some alcohol: longer bleeding, the blood of a light color, red and thin, inflammation, pain, pussing for several days, and healing only after a two days' fasting.

I have offered myself, of course in vain, to the Prussian Ministry of War for a repetition of this experiment. Why is it that the wounds of the Japanese healed much quicker and better in the Russo-Japanese war than those of the "Meat and Brandy Russians"? Has nobody for 2,000 years ever thought it over why the opening of the artery and even the poison cup could not kill Seneca, after he had despised meat and fasted in prison? It is said that even before that, Seneca fed on nothing but fruit and water.

All disease is finally nothing else but a clogging up of the smallest blood vessels, the capillaries, by mucus. Nobody will want to clean the water conduit of a city, a pipe system, which is fed with soiled water by a pump, the filters of which are clogged up, without having the water-supply shut off during the cleaning process. If the conduit supplies the entire city or a portion of it with unclean water, or if even the smallest branch-pipes are clogged up, there is no man in the world who would repair or improve that respective spot; everybody thinks at once of the central, of the tank and the filters, and these together with the pumping machine can be cleaned only as long as the water supply is shut off.

"I am the Lord, thy physician" — English and modern: nature alone heals, cleans, "unmucuses" best and infallibly sure, but only if the supply, or at least the mucus supply, is stopped. Each "physiological machine," man like beast, cleanses itself immediately, dissolves the mucus in the clogged-up vessels, without stopping short as soon as the supply of compact food at least, is interrupted. Even in the case of the supposedly healthy man this mucus, as already mentioned then appears in the urine where it can be seen after cooling off in the proper glass tubes! Whoever denies, ignores or fights this uniform fact, because perhaps, it is not in accord with his teachings, or is not sufficiently scientific, is jointly guilty of the impossibility of detection of the principal cause of all diseases, and this in the first place, to his own detriment.

Therewith I also uncover the last secret of consumption. Or does anybody believe that this enormous quantity of mucus thrown off by a patient stricken with tuberculosis for years and years emanates only from the lung itself? Just because this patient is then almost forcibly fed on "mucus" (pap, milk, fat meats) the mucus can never cease until the lung itself decays and the "bacilli" make their appearance when death becomes inevitable. The mystery of the bacilli is solved simply thus: The gradual clogging up of the blood vessels by mucus leads to decomposition, to fermentation of these mucus products and "boiled, dead-food" residues. These decay partially on the living body (pussy abcesses, cancer, tuberculosis, syphilis, lupus, etc.). Now everybody knows that meat, cheese and all organic matter will again "germinate, put forth bacilli" during the process of decomposition. It is for this reason that these germs appear and are detectable only in the more advanced stage of the disease, when, however, they are not the cause but the product of the disease, and disease-furthering only in so far as the decomposition, for instance, of the lung, is being hastened by them, because the excretions of the bacilli, their toxines, act poisoning. If it be correct that bacilli invade, "infect" from the exterior, then it is nothing but the mucus which makes possible their activity, and furnishes the proper soil; the "disposition."

As already stated, I have repeatedly (once for two years) lived mucusless, i.e., on fruit exclusively. I was no longer in need of a handkerchief which product of civilization I hardly need even up to this date. Has anyone ever seen a healthy animal living in freedom, expectorate or blow its nose? A chronic inflammation of the kidneys, considered deadly, which I was stricken with, was not only healed, but I am enjoying a degree of health and efficiency which by far surpasses even that of my healthiest youth. I want to see the man who, being sick unto death at 31; who can run for two hours and a quarter without a stop, or make an endurance march of 56 hours' duration — eight years later.

It is surely theoretically correct that man was a mere fruit eater in times gone by, and biologically correct, that he can be it even today. Or can the horse-sense of man not conceive without any direct proofs, of the fact that man, before becoming a hunter, lived on fruits only? I even maintain that he did live in absolute health, beauty and strength without pain and grief just the way the Bible says. Fruit only, the sole "mucusless" food, is natural. Everything prepared by man, or supposedly improved by him, is evil. The arguments regarding fruit are scientifically exact; in the apple or banana, for instance, everything can be found contained what man needs. Man is so perfect that he can live on one kind of fruit only, at least for quite some time. This has been conclusively proven by the Mono-diet system of August Engelhardt who solved by his great philosophy and practice of natural life all problems of mankind. But a self-evident truth preached by nature must not be discarded just because no one has been able to apply it in actual practice on account of civilizational considerations. From the eating of fruit only, one gets first a crisis, i.e., cleansing. No man would have ever believed me, that it is possible to live without food for 126 days, in which 49 were undertaken at a stretch, during a period covering 14 months. Now I have done it, and yet this truth is not being understood. Hitherto I state and will teach only this fact, that fruit is the most natural "healing remedy." Whether my calculation is correct will be proven by the next epidemic. I take, however this opportunity to uncover the reasons why the self-evident is not believed in. When in the previous century someone talked about the possibility of phoning from London to Paris, everybody laughed because there had never been such a thing. Natural food is not being believed in any more, because almost no one practices it and living in to-day's civilization, we cannot easily practice it. It must also be considered that contra-interests fear that the prices of other, artificial foodstuffs may drop, and others fear that the food-physiology may receive a shock and physicians become unnecessary. But it is just this fasting and fruit cure which requires very strict observation and instruction — therefore: more doctors and less patients who, however, will gladly pay more if they get well. Thus, the social question regarding doctors is solved — an assertion already made by me publicly in Zurich several years ago.

Almost all fasting attempts fail through ignorance of the fact that with the beginning of the mucusless diet the old mucus is being excreted so much more forcibly until that person is absolutely clean and healthy. THUS THE SEEMINGLY MOST HEALTHY PERSON HAS FIRST TO PASS THROUGH A CONDITION OF SICKNESS (CLEANSING), or go through an intermediate stage of illness to a higher level of health.

This is the "great-cliff" around which so few Vegetarians have failed to go — discarding the basic truth just like the mass of people are doing. I have proven this fact in the "Vegetarische Warte" completely on the basis of experiments and facts; and refuting their greatest objection, that of undernourishment, by an actual fasting experiment of 49 days; with a preceding fruit diet. My state of health was greatly improved thru this radical excretion of mucus, disregarding a few unhygienic circumstances during the test. I received numerous letters of appreciation, especially from the educated classes. The mass of adherents of vegetarianism "mucuses" gaily ahead. Contrasting herewith it can only be said that the poisons (so-called by them): meat, alcohol, coffee and tobacco are in the long run comparatively harmless, AS LONG AS THEY ARE USED MODERATELY.

In order to avoid misunderstanding on the part of teetotalers and vegetarians, I must insert here a few explanations. Meat is not a foodstuff but only a stimulant which ferments, decays in the stomach, the process of decay, however, does not begin in the stomach, but at once after the slaughtering. This has already been proven on living persons by Prof. Dr. S. Graham, and I complete this fact by saying that meat acts as a stimulant just by means of these poisons of decay, and therefore is being erroneously regarded as a strengthening foodstuff. Or is there anyone who can show me chemico-physiologically that the albumen molecule going through the process of decay is being newly reformed in the stomach and celebrates its resurrection in some muscle of the human body? Like alcohol, the meat produces in the beginning stimulating strength and energy until the entire organism is penetrated by it and the break-down inevitable. All the other stimulants act likewise. This, therefore, is a false delusion.

The fundamental evil of all non-vegetaric forms of diet consist always in the overeating of meat, as it is the origin of all the other evils, especially in the craving for alcohol. If fruit is eaten almost exclusively, the eagerness for cup or glass loses itself to chastise himself against it, simply because meat produces the demon thirst. Alcohol is a proven kind of antidote for meat, and the gourmand of the big city, who eats practically nothing but meat, must therefore have wines, Mocha and Havana, in order to at least in some way counteract the heavy meat-poisoning. It is a well-known fact, that, after an opulent dinner, one feels decidedly fresher, physically and mentally, if the stimulants, poisonous in themselves, are taken moderately rather than to stuff one's self full with the "good-eating" to the very fatigue.

I ABSOLUTELY DECLARE WAR ON MEAT AND ALCOHOL; through fruit and moderate eating these great evils are radically diminished. But whoever finds it impossible to entirely give up meat and alcohol is, if he takes them moderately, still far ahead of the vegetaric "over or excess eater". The American, Fletcher proved this most evidently by his tremendous success, and his secret is explained by my experiments which show that a person becomes most efficient and develops best in health if he eats as little as possible! Are not the oldest people as a rule the poorest? Have not the greatest discoverers and inventors sprung from proverty, i.e., been "little eaters"? Were not the greatest of mankind; the prophets, founders of religions, etc., ascetics? Is that culture, to dine excellently thrice a day, and is it social progress that each working-man eats five times a day and then pumps himself full with beer at night? If the sick organism can regenerate by eating nothing, I think the logical consequence is that a healthy organism needs but little food in order to remain healthy, strong and persevering.

All so-called miracles of the saints have their only origin in ascetics, and are today impossible but for the simple reason that, although much praying is done, no fasting is adhered to. This is the only solution of this quarrel. We have no more miracles because we have no more saints, i.e., sanctified and healed by ascetics and fastings. The saints were self-shining, expressed in modern language: medial or radioactive, but only because through asceticism, they were "godly" healthy, and not "by special grace." I just wish to mention here that I myself have succeeded in visible, electric effluences, but only by external and internal sun-energies (sun-baths and food from the "sun-kitchen," fruit).

The entire world is quarreling now regarding these questions and miracles. And here is the solution on the basis of experiments which everybody can repeat if he is brave enough. But it is apparently easier to write books, preach and pray, or to say that I am an exception. This is true, but only so far as pluck and understanding are concerned. Physiologically all men are equal, and whoever cannot be moderate may learn it from me if he wishes to be a real searcher after health.

If a man eats little and is healthy he can, for quite a length of time, digest the most absurd food, meat and starch (mucus), i.e., he can again excrete it. Naturally, he becomes and remains still more perfect and clean if he eats but little fruit, and of this he needs the least because it is the most perfect food. This eternal truth by natural law, man of today will and cannot admit, and has a well-founded fear of it, because he is built up of dead-boiled food and his cells die off and are excreted as soon as he takes his sunbaths, fasts or eats the living cells of fruit. But this cure must be done with the greatest care. The duty of medicine is to protect man from a breakdown of his cells, to hold him above water as long as this is possible only to cause him to die of the disease so much more promptly and quickly which today is fervently wished for. Vegetarianism cannot deny that the consumers of meat and alcohol can also boast of much health and great deeds and high age but taken individually and as a people only so long as but little is eaten and no over-nourishment caused. Eating "too much" takes less revenge in case of meat-eating because meat contains proportionally less "mucus" than starch containing, "mucus" vegetaric food and the celebrated vegetaric dinners with entirely too many dishes daily. I myself have not cared for many years for any meals; I eat only when I have appetite and then so little that it does not cause any harmful effect, if, on account of an experiment, I am obliged to eat something which in itself is not entirely free from objection.

If the most serious diseases can be cured by fasting—which has been proven in thousands of cases—and if during the fast one becomes stronger "if it is done right," then the most energetic food, the fruit, should cause one so much the more to become strong and healthy. This has also been scientifically proven by the merited Dr. Bircher. It is true, the science of cure by nature has recognized the fact that something must get out of the sick organism, but it has so far ascribed the greatest importance to physical stimulations ignoring completely the real natural moment to the process of cure; the abstaining from food and thru following a fruit-diet. At least, they have only offered a substitute by a non-alcohol and meatless diet. This does not mean much in the face of my "mucus-theory." And what is this mucusless alcohol not accused of today? It will soon be made the "scape-goat" of all diseases, because here and there is found a depraved one who, consuming it in enormous quantities, ends in delirium. Just compel a drinker to fast a few days or to eat nothing but fruit—I will wager that the best glass of beer will have lost its flavor for him. This proves that the entire "civilized" mess, from beefsteak down to apparently harmless oatmeals, creates the desire for these detested antidotes: alcohol, coffee, tea, tobacco. Why? **Because much-eating paralyzes and only the use of stimulants restores!**

Here is the true and fundamental reason for the increase of alcohol consumption: the over-nourishment, especially with meat. Prof. Dr. Graham says in his "Physiology of Nourishment": "A drinker can reach a high age, a glutton never." This is true, because the acute alcohol acts as a stimulant; and especially the modern beer is less harmful in the long run than the chronic stuffing up of the digestive channel with mucus forming food.

I now ask: what appeals more to reason—to wipe out the masses of mucus, piled up since childhood, or having infected the cellular tissues of the body by poisonous Drugs, or parts cut away by useless, avoidable operations; having the cure delayed by one-sided Osteopathy; Chiropractic malpractice misunderstood Electrical treatments, mucus forming and often unclean milk cures, weakening Hot Springs treatments; the Christian Science superstition, etc., or simply to stop the further supply of mucus caused by unnatural Diet? Or is there anybody who would like to prove to me that the most skillful Chef or Confectioner is capable of producing something better than an apple, a grape or banana? If nourishment by mucus and over-eating is the true fundamental cause of all diseases without exception, which I can prove to anybody on his own body, then there can exist but one natural remedy, i.e., fasting and fruit-diet. That every animal fasts in case of even the slightest uneasiness, is a well-known fact and to culture and thanks to man feeding them, domestic animals have lost their sharp instinct for the right kind of food and the natural hours of feeding—and therewith their proper state of health and acuteness of sense—they will never-the-less when sick, accept only the most necessary food; they fast themselves back to health. Poor, sick man, however, must under no circumstances live on short rations for more than 1 or 2 days, for fear that he may "lose strength."

Already many leading physicians have called fasting: wonder cures, cure of the uncured, cure of all cures, etc. Certain charlatans have brought this infallible, but at the same time, dangerous cure, to discredit. I have done in fasting the most significant thing in centuries: 49 days, world-record (see "Vegetarsche Warte," 1909, book 19, 20, 22, 1920, book 1 and 2). Furthermore I am the only one who combines this cure with systematically and individually adapted fruit diet, which makes it astonishingly easier and absolutely harmless. We are, therefore, undoubtedly put in a position to heal diseases which the school of medicine designates as incurable. On the basis of my deduction that this mucus coming from cultured food, is the fundamental cause and main factor in the nature of all diseases, symptoms of age, obesity, falling out of the hair, wrinkles, weakness of nerves and memory, etc., there is justified hope for the creation of a new phase of development of the progressive healing methods and biological medicine.

Already Hippokrates had uniformly recognized the "disease-material" for all diseases. Prof. Jaeger has defined the "Common" as "Stench," but had not discovered the source of this "bad smell." Dr. Lahmann and other representatives of the physical dietetic tendency, especially Kuhne, came on to the tracks of the "common foreign matter." But not one of them showed, recognized or proved by experiment, that it is this very mucus of culture-food which loads up our organism from childhood, and attacks it at a certain degree of fermentation, forms pathologic beds, i.e., decomposes the cellular tissue of the body itself into pus and decay. It is being mobilized in case of casual colds or high temperatures, etc., and produces, in its tendency to leave the body, symptoms of abnormal functions which hitherto have been regarded as the disease itself. It is, therefore, for the first time possible to define what is meant by "decomposition." The more the "mucus" (bad mother's milk and all its substitutes) is being administered from childhood on, or the less this mucus is being excreted, owing to hereditary weakness, through the organs made to perform this task, the greater is the inclination to catch cold, fever, to freeze, to admit parasites, to get sick and to pre-maturely grow old. Very likely by this the veil has been lifted from the secret which hitherto has always surrounded the nature of the white corpuscles. I believe that here, as in many other cases, we are confronted with an error of medical science. The bacteria throw themselves upon the white corpuscles, composed to the largest extent of this mucus; denounced by me. Are not the bacteria being bred on this mucus by the millions outside of the organism?—on potatoes, broth, gelatine, i.e., on mucus, i.e., nitrogenous, vegetable or animal substances consisting of an alkalically reacting fluid containing granulated cells of the appearance of the white blood-corpuscles? Perhaps in an entirely healthy condition the so-called mucus membrane should not at all be white, slimy, but clean and red like on animals. Perhaps this "corpse-mucus" is even the cause of the paleness of the white race! Paleface! Corpsecolor!

With this "mucus-theory" to be confirmed by experiment the spectre "disease" has been finally deprived of its demoniac mask. He who believes me can heal not only himself, if everything else fails, but we have for the first time been given the means to radically prevent disease and to make it definitely impossible. Even the dream of lasting youth and beauty is now about to become true.

The animal, and especially the human organism, is, from a mechanical standpoint, a complicated tube-system of blood-vessels with air-gas impetus by means of the lungs in which the blood-fluid is constantly kept moving and regulated by the heart as a valve. The decomposition of the air-gas is accomplished by each breath in the lungs (separating of the air into oxygen and nitrogen): thus the blood is constantly kept moving and the human body does its service incredibly long without fatigue. Let nobody come to me with the silly excuse of the "daily experience of the absolutely natural compulsion of much-eating," prescribed for working man, etc., before it has not been experienced by such complainant, how long it is possible to work or march, without fatigue, after fasting or fruit-food. Fatigue is in the first place a reducing of strength by too much digestion-work, secondly a clogging-up of the heated and consequently narrowed-down blood-vessels, and thirdly a "self-and re-poisoning" through the excretion of mucus during the motion. All organic substances of animal origin excrete cyanate groupes in their decomposition, which the chemist Hensel has defined as bacilli proper. The air is not only the highest ,and most perfect operating material of the human body, but simultaneously the first element for the erection, repair, substitute, and very likely, the animal organism derives nitrogen also from the air. On certain caterpillars an increase of weight through air alone has been stated.

Complete Fasting, - followed by a decrease in the quantity of food eaten, is the only check on "over-eating". And a diet of "non-mucus-forming" foods must replace the "mucus-forming" foods. Fresh tree-ripened fruits and the green-leaf starchless vegetables have been long recognized and my Mucusless Diet Healing System is already a well proven fact! Neither fasting nor the fruit diet have been accepted by the medical authorities nor have they been used by others in strict accordance with the condition of the patient; yet when properly combined as a "systematic cleansing", the treatment has been remarkably successful and satisfactory. The degree of the individuals weakness, together with the disturbing sensations, experienced by the patient are an extremely important factor that must be given full consideration. My cure is the only one on record, that can be regulated and controlled as to speed!

Remedies for the Removal of the Common Fundamental Cause of Diseases and the Prevention of Their Re-occurrence

After having told my readers the dread and horror of being sick or getting sick, in the previous chapter, it befits me to show them the means and ways, as far as this, commonly speaking, is possible, how to successfully encounter mucus-poisoning, this greatest foe of health. Here I wish to show three means and ways which can produce a beneficial change.

1. The shortest and best way is the fasting so much talked about in this book. It cuts short the life of the "grim misdoer" in our body and causes him to flee, and he leaves us faster with fright and terror.

Healthy people can submit themselves to a fasting cure without any further ceremony. It goes without saying that they must fast reasonably and assume personal responsibility, and not cause dangerous over-exertions during the fasting period, by demanding of themselves physical or mental performances which they could not live up to even at full fare. I insert here a precautionary measure which must be observed in all fasting cures; the complete emptying of the bowels at the beginning of the fasting by harmless purgative (such as an aromatic herb compound), or by a syringe, or by both. It lies in the nature of the thing that he who fasts must not be bothered by gas or decomposing matter which form from the excrements remaining in the bowels; it suffices that the mucus during the excretion gives him enough trouble, as already stated.

If it is not desired to take a more prolonged fast, although he is healthy, one should try a short one. Even a fasting of thirty-six hours, weekly one or two times, can be depended upon to produce very favorable results. It is best to start by leaving off the supper and taking an enema instead.

Then, in the case of a thirty-six hours' fast, nothing is eaten until the following morning, the meal to consist of nothing but fruits. The eating of fruit is desirable after each fasting, as the juices of the fruits cause a moving of the mucus-masses, which have loosened. However let me caution all; especially the sick and elderly people; this treatment must be carefully individualized.

One arrives at this result much sooner, however, if a longer fasting is done in the way described, for instance, three days, and then continue what I call an after-fasting cure. That is, do not eat anything for three days and drink only fresh lemonade, unsugared, in single gulps as may become necessary, and begin on the fourth day with some fruits. At the close of the fourth day take a thorough enema. More fruit may be added from day to day, until about the seventh day of the "after-cure" the normal quantity of fruit-diet in the proper composition and selection has been reached. The fasting, however, can be extended for weeks by healthy persons and by those whose occupation permits of their spending their time in bed in case of difficult excretions of mucus. Nobody should seriously object to the so-called "bad looks" or the decrease in weight. The body fasts itself into health, despite the miserable complexion, and in a remarkably short time the cheeks will be adorned by a healthy, natural red. The weight is also restored to its normal standard very soon after the fasting. After a fast the body reacts on every ounce of food. Very moderate eaters and frequently fasting people have a very fine, spiritual expression of the face. It is said that Pope Leo XIII, that great faster and life-artist, had a very clear, almost transparent complexion.

In this connection I wish to call attention to another point, already mentioned elsewhere, for the success of the fasting depends upon it to a great extent. The fasting person must not unnecessarily become depressed or ill-humored; the one condition finds relief in the disagreeable moments by complete rest, the other by quick and decided work, especially in light and mechanical occupation.

When the body has been ridden of the mucus, slime and paste, then it is the sacred duty of the person who has regained health to keep up the reclaimed highest earthly happiness and to guard it by means of natural, correct food. On this subject a few short remarks in the following paragraphs will not come amiss.

2. He who cannot fast, because of considerations of advanced lung or heart trouble, for instance, may at least see to it that the further accumulation of mucus be cut short by refraining from pronounced mucus-formers, especially from all flour (cake), rice, potato dishes, boiled milk, cheese, meat, etc. Whoever cannot miss bread entirely, must eat black or white bread only toasted; by toasting, the bread loses much of its harmfulness, as the mucus substances are partly destroyed. The eating of toasted bread or whole wheat Zweiback has the further advantage that not much can be eaten of it; it cannot be devoured as wild beasts do, and the necessary chewing

will fatigue even the most greedy gums. Whoever cannot bite the toasted bread, on account of bad teeth, may suck on it until it dissolves—a splendid way to restore declined strength. Whoever cannot miss potatoes should eat them only baked, and be sure and eat the jackets.

What then remains for "nutritious food" after I am to give up all albuminous food, like dried peas, lentils, beans, as much as possible? Thus many a reader will ask with a sigh.

As to the value of meat I have set forth my views elsewhere. The slight requirements in albumen are fully covered by sugary fruits; the banana, the nuts, combined with a few figs or dates are first class muscle-formers and strength-givers.

The vegetable (cut small and made into salad), the salads themselves, prepared with oil and plenty of fresh lemon juice, and all the splendid fruits and berries, including those of the South, are worthy of being served on the tables of Gods. And when springtime comes, and last season's fruits, especially apples are on the decline, and the new vegetables not yet ready, does not Mother Nature help us out abundantly with oranges from the South? Will the aroma and wealth of these splendid products of nature not induce man to eventually become a fruit-eater entirely?

It is not possible for me to go into the question of food and its effects exhaustively in this book; for healthy people these statements may suffice; to sick people I recommend special prescriptions according to their state of health. If you are not already an owner of my Mucusless Diet Healing System Lesson Course may I suggest that you secure a copy of this book. It may be mentioned that non-fasters and people easily succumbing to illness, may at least follow the morning's fastings, or non-breakfast plan. It would be better for all concerned not to eat anything before 10 o'clock AM and then nothing but fruits. The reward for this little self-chastising will certainly show itself shortly—especially if the latter be kept up unfailingly.

3. Now, just one more word to those who think it impossible to give up the accustomed mucus food (meat, bread, etc.). To those "unfortunate ones" I give this advice: Chew each bite of your food thoroughly; as recommended by the American Fletcher, in one word, "Fletcherize." Not that the fruit eaters should over-look this; but certainly the poison-laden "mucus-eaters" must do so; especially if they do not wish to sink into their graves all too soon.

The strong secretion of saliva in slow chewing decreases the formation of mucus and helps to prevent overeating. Of course, this group of individuals cannot expect to achieve in health and strength; retain youth and perseverance; physical and mental efficiency, as achieved by the faster and fruiteater! Once man is healthy in my sense of the word, thru fasting and fruit diet; that is; free from mucus, slime and germs, and if he continues on the fruit-diet, he, of course, need not fast any longer; for only then will he find pleasure in eating which he never dreamt of before. Only in this way will man find the way to happiness, harmony and the solution of all health problems. Only through following this diet can man become want-free and get "nearest to divinity."

The Fundamental Cause of Growing Old and Ugly

THE MEANS FOUNDED IN NATURE FOR MAINTENANCE OF YOUTH AND BEAUTY

Following the previous general arguments to the effect that mucus is the main cause of disease and ageing, there is only left to show in particular and on the various organs, in how far the mucus of culture-food acts "beauty-hindering" in the construction of the human body, and produces symptoms of ugliness and age.

If, according to paradisaic primary laws, the lungs and skin would be given nothing but pure air and sun-electricity, and the stomach and bowels nothing but sun-food, i.e., fruits, which are being digested almost without rest, secreting only mucusless, pasteless and germless cellulose, there seems to be no reason why the tube-system of the human body should become defective, weaken, age and finally break down entirely. Instead of the living energy-cells of the fruit, one eats "killed food," which biologically is meant for beasts of prey, i.e., food chemically changed by air-oxidation (decay), dead-boiled and robbed of its energy. Mucus accumulates especially in the heating channel (stomach and bowels) of the tube-machine, and slowly clogs up the channel and filters (glands). The sum-total of this defilement causes chronic defects, makes one grow old and is the main factor in the nature of all disease. Growing old, therefore, is actually a latent disease, that is, a slow but constantly increasing disturbance in the operation of the motor of life.

The chemistry of victuals gives the most reliable proof that deformity and decomposition have their source mainly in the lack of minerals in boiled culture-food.

If human ugliness as such, lost beauty and symptoms of growing old can be made accountable for by wrong nourishment, then the theory of beauty and rejuvenation leads to a dietetic cure and a respective improvement of nourishment. But inasmuch as beauty, especially human beauty, cannot be absolutely defined, because everybody has a different taste, I can limit myself only to the main standards of aesthetic demands.

The white corpse-color of the light and sunless man of culture cannot be considered beautiful; since it emanates mainly from the white corpse-color of the dead-boiled, wrong food. What wonderful color a man can get who feeds on "bleeding" grapes, cherries and oranges and who systematically takes air and sun-baths; cannot be imagined by the modern artists of "pleinair-painting." Mucus and at the same time lack of mineral matter means as much as lack of color. Just compare the food tables of Dr. Konig and you will find that the mucusless food; the fruits and starchless greenleaf vegetables, occupy the first place as regards their contents of necessary mineral matter, especially lime. The size of a person, i.e., the circumference of the skeleton, depends for instance, mainly on the amount of lime contained in the food. The Japanese want to increase the size of their race by meat, thereby going from bad to worse. All the pining away of size; deformities of the bones, and faulty vision and decay of the teeth, is due to lack of lime. Through the boiling of milk and vegetables in modern cooking the lime content is being eliminated. The enormous poorness in minerals of cultured-food, especially of the meat as compared with fruit, is responsible for the coming of a toothless human race, as predicted even by physicians, and which is not merely a phantom of imagination. And instead of by fruit these stuffs are being substituted by an organic preparation. The human organism does not assimilate one single atom of mineral substance which has not transmigrated into a plant of fruit, i.e., which has not become organic. The most modern disfigurement, the obesity, has clouded up our aesthetic feeling in this regard so much that we even do not know any longer the limit of the normal. I personally do not even consider the physical culturist "man of muscles of classic type" beautiful and as a standard for the ideal type of Germanic and Aryan races. Weight, shape and especially circumference of body are too great. Every accumulation of fat is pathologic and in this measure unaesthetic. No animal living in freedom is upholstered with fat, like our modern "weight lifters and strong men." The reason is simply too much food and too much fluid; relaxation and clogging of the entire system of vessels are the natural consequences. Grape-sugar of the fruits and their nutritive salts are the right sources for a firm muscle-substance, by which a body disfattened and dis-mucused by fasting can be quickly rebuilt.

The stoutness of face and body are dangerously on the increase; it is ugly and certainly pathologic. It is a curious fact that in our supposedly enlightened age this accumulation of fat is considered not only beautiful, but even a sign of overabundant health, while the daily experience teaches that the slim, permanently youthful type possesses in every respect a greater force of resistance and generally reaches greater longevity.

I should like to be shown just one person of 90 or 100 years with such obesity, which today is pronounced as beautiful and healthy, and with which it is believed to fatten away tuberculosis. If fat people do not die in their best years through palpitation of the heart, apoplexy or dropsy, they succumb to a slow emaciating and the desire for food decreases in spite of all artificial stimulations of the appetite. The skin, especially of the face, having been subjected to extreme tension, becomes foldy and wrinkly. It has lost its youthful elasticity on account of insufficient and unhealthy blood circulation as well as lack of light and sun. And now this relaxation of the skin is being tried to be prevented by salves and powders applied externally! The distinction and beauty of the features, the pureness and healthy color of the complexion, the clearness and natural size of the eyes, the charm of the expression and the color of the lips, age and become ugly to the extent of the expression and color of the mucus in the bowels, which we have recognized above as the central depot from which all the symptoms of diseases, and therefore those of age, are being fed. The "beautiful roundness of cheeks" which at the same time increases the size of the nose, is nothing but a clogging up by mucus, which, as is well known, breaks out in case of a cold in the nose.

The Preservation of the Hair

REASONS FOR BECOMING BALD AND GRAY

I come now to the most important and most striking symptom of the growing-old: the falling out and getting gray of the hair, to which I must devote an entire section, because its appearance generally causes the first and greatest worry and pain over the coming of age, and because hitherto science has stood baffled in the face of this problem.

The modern cutting short of the feminine as well as the masculine hair on the head, and the alarming expansion and earliness of baldness have accustomed even an artistical eye so much to this appearance that we no longer become conscious of the fact of how seriously the aesthetic and harmonic figure of man is disturbed by the voluntary and involuntary "hair-decapitation." Man who is not only intellectual, but also is an aesthetic product of nature, "the crown of creation," is being robbed of the splendid crown of his head—the hair. They could be called "living skulls," these beardless, colorless and expressionless heads of today! Just imagine the most beautiful woman with a pate! Where is the man that would not turn away with horror? Or a fashion-sport of today hewn in marble! In addition to that the mustache shaped geometrically and angular or trimmed off entirely, then the modern clothing which distinguishes itself from that of all the centuries by the greatest insipidity—and this we find beautiful reasons, for which the present-day man gets his beard removed and his hair cut down to a minimum length. The lack of beauty and therewith the unaesthetic appearance of hair and beard has become so general that in course of time the need of shaving and use of the clipper have come as a matter of course. In our time of equalization and all-leveling it is preferred, and rightfully so, to cut off these odor, and so to speak, revelation-organs of inner man, instead of furnishing by ugly, disheveled, uneven and hereditary morbid hair, a living proof for the descendants theory. Therewith we can understand the maltreatment of the hair. The thought has practically given rise that the getting ugly of one organ or of the entire organism means its inner morbidness, i.e., nature reveals internal physiological disturbances of an organism through disharmony of shape and color. The seriously ill and dead organism are its extremes. Doubters of my point of view, and bad nature-observers may here be reminded of the law of exception from the rule, and as regards man—of the fact, that neither hygienically nor aesthetically have we any imagination left of the ideal beauty and health of man living under perfectly natural conditions. If the pleasure in the beautiful is a sentence in the favorable sense, then the displeasure felt by an aesthetic eye in looking upon the disharmony of shape and color must include to a certain degree the recognition of the pathologic.

Let us return to our subject. We know that medical science is powerless as regards baldness, and that cosmetics and chemistry of tonics have failed to produce even a single new hair.

I have already called the hair, especially of the human head, the odor-organs of the body, which are to conduct away the exhalations of the human body. Everybody knows that sweat is produced first of all on the head and in the arm-pits, and that with this sweat, especially on sick people, is connected a disagreeable odor. Dr. Jaeger calls disease somewhere "stench." This, with exceptions, of course, seems to me correct in so far as I am able to pronounce, on the basis of many years' observation and experiments, the following fundamental uniform conception of disease:

Disease is a fermentation and decay-process of body-substance or of surplus and unnatural food-material which in course of time has accumulated, especially in the digestive organs, and which makes its appearance in the shape of mucus-excretion.

That is, it means in the last instance nothing but the chemical decomposition, the decay of cellular albumen. As is well known, this process is accompanied by stench, while nature combines the originating of new life with fragrance (the building of plants). Properly, man in perfect health should exhale fragrance, particularly so with his hair. Poets are rightfully comparing man with a flower and speak of the hairfragrance of woman. I, THEREFORE, RECOGNIZE IN THE HAIR OF THE HUMAN A VERY IMPORTANT ORGAN WHICH ASIDE FROM PROTECTIVE AND WARMTH-REGULATING PURPOSES HAS A HIGHLY INTERESTING AND USEFUL DESTINATION: to conduct away the exhalations, the odor of healthy and sick people, which reveals to experts and acute noses not only individual qualities, but even certain disclosures as regards the inner state of health or sickness of a man. If the doctors have not by far recognized digestive disturbances with the microscopes and test glasses, there have yet been certain quacks who have been able to state by simple hairdiagnosis the stench-producing inner process of decay — the disease. Why, there are numberless people today, still youthful and radiating health with a breath like that of a sewer and who are wondering why their hair is falling out.

I have now arrived at the vital spot of my researches and observations.

First one more word about the getting gray of the hair. It has been found that in hair which has become gray the contents of air is increasing, and I am also of the opinion that this "air" consists probably of stinking gases, or at least is mixed with such. I recommend to a chemist with a "strong scent" to discover here the sulphurous acid, then the disappearance of the color of the hair will also have been explained, as it is a well-known fact that sulphur-dioxide bleaches organic substances.

It now seems to me certain, not only theoretically, but also on the basis of my interesting experiments on my own body, that the principal cause of baldness can only be an internal one. If through these odor-tubes or so to speak, "gas chimneys of the head," there must be constantly discharged stinking, corroding gases, very probably impregnated with sulphur-dioxide, instead of natural, fragrant odors, we must not be surprised if the hair together with its roots becomes deathly pale, dies off and falls out. Herewith I claim to have recognized the reason for baldness and to have shown the true way for its cure. I add that about ten years ago, when I was afflicted with chronic inflammation of the kidneys, combined with a high degree of nervosity, my hair had become very gray and fell out. After having been cured from this serious disease by a dietetic treatment I saw that at the same time the gray hairs disappeared and that my hair grew into perfect profusion.

If, therefore, the main cause of baldness lies in the disturbance of digestion and interchange of matter, it can certainly be cured by regulation of these functions. It can be said that even the absolutely bald heads may again take hope, on the basis of my discovery — after all the tonics have failed, and must fail. The reason is that the cause is not external and therefore cannot be got at externally. Whoever sees his hair falling out, or whoever is already bald, and wishes to regenerate in this direction, may apply to me for advice. There is no general internal remedy, and whoever has understood me will appreciate that individualization is necessary in every case. On the basis of the influence of my doctrine of diet on digestion, and creation of clean, pure blood, supplying the correct nourishment of the hair-bed, I can at least guarantee a standstill of the falling out of hair, if my advice is followed correctly.

Thus, all symptoms of ageing are latent disease, accumulation of mucus and clogging-up by mucus. Everybody subjecting himself to a thorough restoring-cure in case of any disease, by parting with the dead cells, through mucusless diet and eventually fasting, rejuvenates himself simultaneously, and whoever submits to a rejuvenating cure, deprives each and every disease of its foundation. Nobody wants to believe in this possibility. Yet, in each scientific dictionary you will find the theory that at the worst one should die only of disturbance in the exchange of matter, i.e., constipation by mucus, so that life ought to end without any disease whatever. This would be the normal; but, alas, the exception — the disease, has become the rule today.

IF ANYBODY WOULD LIVE FROM CHILDHOOD, ON ABSOLUTELY MUCUSLESS FOOD, AND FEED ON NOTHING BUT FRUIT, IT WOULD BE JUST AS CERTAIN THAT HE COULD GROW NEITHER OLD NOR SICK. I have seen persons who through a mucusless cure have rejuvenated and become beautiful to such an extent that they could not be recognized. Since thousands of years humanity dreams, imagines and paints the fountain of youth, and looks for it sentimentally to the stars, in the suggestion.

Think of the amounts being expended for remedies for masculine weakness and impotence, for sterility — of course all in vain! And how easy it would be to help some people; especially through correct and nourishing food from the sun-kitchen.

We cannot imagine with what beauty and faculties the paradisiacal "godlike" man was gifted, what wonderful strong, clear voice he had! The beautification and strengthening of the voice, yes, the winning back of the lost voice, is an amazing symptom in my cure, and especially eloquent proof for the really grandiose effect of my system for the entire organism of the patient. I wish to refer here especially to the wonderful success of the cure submitted to by the Royal Bavarian Chamber Singer Heinrich Knote, Munich, under my directions, whose voice had improved to the amazement of the entire musical world.

Increasing Longevity

In the previous chapters I have quoted the clogging-up by mucus as being the reason for disease and ageing. I have also proved the possibility of re-substitution of dead-cells. In view of the latter fact it cannot be denied that the entire standstill of the human motor can be delayed for a long, long time, if the body is being built up and maintained by living sun-food from childhood on. At any rate the body thus nourished is far ahead of that of the wrong food and "all-eater" in that its building material is much more durable. In the right way of living the exchange of matter takes place to a much lesser degree, likewise the stress on the inner organs, especially the heart and the stomach. In the performance of greatest efforts the mucusless organism has not nearly the pulse-frequency of a "much-eater." Merely through this saving of energy it is possible to mathematically figure out and prove an advantage as regards longevity. But can we perhaps even solve by this all-explaining mucus-constipation the last of all mysteries—death?

In life-endangering injuries and afflictions the brain and the heart are the organs whose disturbance of function finally ends with death. We can say that in most diseases death takes place through additional development of heart-illness. As regards this, science has not by far spoken its last word, but we can say that the clogging up of the blood vessels of the heart and the destruction of the tender heart-nerves through permanent re-poisoning of the blood is the final cause of death in all chronic diseases. Likewise the clogging up of the tender blood-vessels in the brain and an eventual bursting of same (apoplexy), as well as any other entire clogging up of vessels to a stand-still of all functions of life produces death. Of course, other circumstances also play a part in it, for instance, insufficient supply of air in case of disease of the lungs. Science also mentions the excessive appearance of the white blood-corpuscles as the reason for death. This process of disease is regarded as a disease in itself, and called "Leukaemia"—white bloodedness, but more proper in my opinion: more mucus than blood. Many other reasons are given for the cause of death.

If, perchance, a disease cannot be put into any of the better defined registers, it is given the name of "cachexy," which sounds very wise but means: bad conditions of nourishment, decay. I now ask, what is really the killing poison? Modern medical science gives the bacilli as the cause for most of the diseases, thus showing that it also has the idea of a common fundamental factor for all diseases, the ageing and death, and undoubtedly a large part of all diseases and their consequences (death) are due to the bacilli. My experimental proof that mucus is the fundamental and main factor differs from the bacillus theory only in that just this mucus is the bed, the pre-condition, the primary.

The excessive appearance of the white blood-corpuscles, i.e., of the white dead mucus, as compared with the red sugar and iron substances, is becoming dangerous to life. Red colored and sweet is the visible token of life and love; white, pale, colorless, bitter; the token of disease and overwhelming by mucus, the slow-dying away of the individual.

The death-struggle or agony can only be regarded as a last crisis, a last effort of the organism to excrete mucus; a last fight of the still living cells against the dead ones and their death-poisons. If the white, dead cells, the mucus in the blood, gain the upper hand, there takes place not only a mechanical clogging-up in the heart, but also a chemical reformation, a decline, a total-poisoning, a sudden decay of the entire blood-supply—and the machine stops short. "It has pleased God Almighty;" "we bend our knees before the mysterious power of death"—thus we speak with resignation.

PART II.
Complete Instructions for Fasting

Most diseases are due to wrong eating habits, incorrect food combinations, acidulous foods and the commercial foods of present day civilization. How to overcome the results of these errors that the majority of us. ignorantly inflict upon ourselves will be taught in the following pages.

For thousands of years Fasting has been recognized as Nature's Supreme curative measure. But the art of When, Why and How to fast has been lost by those living in present day civilization with a very few exceptions. The body must have good nourishing food—is the battle cry of today. But just what is good nourishing food?

The unfortunate sufferers go the rounds of the various schools of therapeutics, some of them deliberate fakirs—others unknowingly ignorant but in the majority of cases groping darkly and in vain for the truth. And the unfortunate part of it all is that they die before they learn the truth. Religious evangelists and divine healers have the advantage of giving Nature a chance—prescription "specialists," scientific surgery—serum injectors and vaccine innoculators are the real offenders of an outraged nature. And so it resolves itself into a case of "blind leading the blind." How simple it is to receive instructions from Nature. Watch the animals heal themselves in time of illness—without the use of so-called scientific medicine. This then is the supreme secret of Mother Nature's Self-healing.

In these chapters we intend showing why it is necessary to use cooked foods as well as natural foods to properly balance your diet. We will also explain the causes of fermentation and gas producing foods.

Rational Fasting for Physical, Mental and Spiritual Rejuvenation

It is significant for our time of degeneration that fasting, by which I mean living without solid and liquid food, is still a problem as a leading factor for the average man, as well as for the orthodox medical doctor. Even Naturopathy required a few decades in its development to take up Nature's only, universal and omnipotent "remedy" of healing. It is further significant that fasting is still considered as a "special" kind of cure, and due to some truly "marvelous" results here and there, it has quite recently become a world-wide fad. Some expert Nature-cure advocators plan-out general "prescriptions" of fasting, and how to break a fast regardless of your condition or the cause from which you are a sufferer.

On the other hand, fasting is so feared and misrepresented that the average man actually considers you a fool if you miss a few meals when sick, thinking you will starve to death, when in reality you are being cured. He fails to understand the difference between fasting and starvation. The medical doctor in general endorses and, in fact, teaches such foolish beliefs regarding Nature's only foundational law of all healing and "curing."

Whatever has been designed and formulated to eliminate the disease matters and designated as "natural treatments" without having at least some restriction or change in diet, or fasting, is a fundamental disregard of the truth concerning the cause of disease.

Have you ever thought what the lack of appetite means when sick? And that animals have no doctors, and no drug stores, and no sanitariums, and no machinery to heal them?

Nature demonstrates and teaches by that example that there is only one disease and that one is caused thru eating—and, therefore, every disease whatsoever it may be named by man, is and can be healed by one "remedy" only—by doing the direct opposite of the cause—by the compensation of the wrong—i.e., reducing the quantity of food or fasting. The reason so many, and especially, long fasting, cures have failed and continue to fail is due to the ignorance which still exists, regarding what is going on in the body during a fast—an ignorance still existing even in the minds of naturopaths and fasting experts up to the present date.

I dare say there may not be another man in history who has studied, investigated, tested and experimented on fasting as much as I did. There is no other expert at present, as far as I know, who conducted so many fasting cures on the most severe cases, as I did. I opened the first special sanitarium in the world for fasting, combined with the Mucusless Diet, and fasting is an essential part of my* Mucusless Diet Healing System. I have likewise made four public scientific tests of fastings of 21, 24, 32 and 49 days, respectively, as a scientific demonstration. The latter test is the world's record of a fast conducted under a strict scientific supervision of government officials.

You may therefore believe me when I teach something new and instructive about what actually happens in the body during a fast. You have learned that the body must be first considered as a machine, a mechanism made of rubber-like material which has been over-expanded during its entire life thru overeating. Therefore, the functioning of the or-

* Prof. Arnold Ehret is the originator of the Mucusless Diet Healing System. These lessons, now available in book form, are published by Ehret Literature Publishing Co., Beaumont, California 92223.

ganism is continually obstructed by an unnatural over-pressure of the blood and on the tissues. As soon as you stop eating, this over-pressure is rapidly relieved, the avenues of the circulation contract, the blood becomes more concentrated and the superfluous water is eliminated. This goes on for the first few days and you may even feel fine, but then the obstructions of the circulation become greater because the diameter of the avenues become smaller and the blood must circulate thru many parts of the body, especially in the tissues, at and around the symptom, against sticky mucus pressed-out and disolved from the inside walls; in other words, the blood stream must overcome, dissolve and carry with itself mucus and poisons for elimination thru the kidneys.

When you fast you eliminate first and at once the primary obstructions of wrong and too much eating. This results in your feeling relatively good, or possibly even better than when eating, but, as previously explained, you bring new, secondary obstructions from your own waste in the circulation and you feel miserable. You and everyone else blames the lack of food. The next day you can notice with certainty mucus in the urine and when the quantity of waste, taken in the circulation, is eliminated, you will undoubtedly feel fine, even stronger than ever before. So it is a well-known fact that a faster can feel better and is actually stronger on the twentieth day than on the fifth or sixth day—certainly a tremendous proof that **vitality does not depend primarily on food,** but rather from an unobstructed circulation. (See Lesson 5 of my Mucusless Diet Healing System.) The smaller the amount of "O" (obstruction) the greater "P" (air pressure) and therefore "V" (vitality).

Thru the above enlightening explanation you see that fasting is—First, a negative proposition to relieve the body from direct obstructions of solid, most unnatural foods; second, that it is a mechanical process of elimination by contracting tissues pressing out mucus, causing friction and obstruction in the circulation.

The following are examples of vitality from "P" Power, air-pressure alone:

One of my first fasters, a relatively healthy vegetarian, walked 45 miles in the mountains on his 24th fast day.

A friend, fifteen years younger, and myself walked 56 HOURS CONTINUALLY after a ten-day fast.

A German physician, a specialist in fasting-cures, published a pamphlet entitled "Fasting, the Increase of Vitality." He learned the same fact that I did, but he does not know why and how, and vitality therefore remained mysterious for him.

If you drink only water, during a fast, the human mechanism cleanses itself, the same as though you would press out a dirty watery sponge, but the dirt in this instance is sticky mucus and in many cases pus and drugs, which must pass thru the circulation until it is so thoroughly dissolved that it can pass thru the fine structure of the "physiological sieve" called kidneys.

Building a Perfect Body Thru Fasting

As long as the waste is in the circulation you feel miserable during a fast; as soon as it is thru the kidneys you feel fine. Two or three days later and the same process repeats itself. It must now be clear to you why conditions change so often during a fast; it must now be clear to you why it is possible for you to feel unusually better and stronger on the twentieth day than on the fifth, for instance.

But this entire cleansing work, thru continued contracting of the tissue (becoming lean) must be done by, and with the original, old blood composition of the patient, and consequently a long fast, especially a too long fast, may become in fact a crime if the sick organism is too greatly clogged up by waste. Fasters who died from too long a fast did not die from lack of food, but actually suffocated in and with their own waste. I made this statement years ago. More clearly expressed: The immediate cause of death is not a poverty of blood in vital substances, but from too much obstruction. "O" (obstruction) becomes as great as or even greater than "P" (air pressure), and the body mechanism is at its "death point."

I GAVE ALL OF MY FASTERS LEMONADE WITH A TRACE OF HONEY OR BROWN SUGAR FOR LOOSENING AND THINNING THE MUCUS IN THE CIRCULATION. Lemon juice and fruit acids of all kinds neutralize the stickiness of mucus and pus (acid paste cannot be used).

If a patient has ever taken drugs over his entire life period —which are stored up in the body like the waste from food, his condition might easily become serious or even dangerous when these poisons enter the circulation, when he takes his first fast. Palpitation of the heart, headaches, nervousness may set in, and especially insomnia. I saw patients eliminate drugs they had taken as long as forty years before. Symptoms such as described above are blamed on the fast by everybody and espcially doctors.

HOW LONG SHOULD ONE FAST?

Nature answers this question in the animal kingdom with a certain cruelty — "fast until you are either healed or dead!" In my estimation 50 to 60% of the so-called "healthy" men of today and 80 to 90% of the seriously chronic sick would die from their latent diseases thru a long fast.

How long one should fast cannot be definitely stated at all, in advance, even in cases where the condition of the patient is known. When and how to break the fast is determined by noting carefully how conditions change during the fast; — you now understand that the fast should be broken as soon as you notice that the obstructions are becoming too great in the circulation, and the blood needs new vital substance to resist and neutralize the poisons.

Change your ideas regarding the claim "the longer you fast the better the cure." You may now readily understand why. Man is the sickest animal on earth; no other animal has violated the laws of eating as much as man; no other animal eats as wrongly as man.

Here is the point where human intelligence can correctively assist in the self-healing process by the following adjustments which embrace the Mucusless Diet Healing System:

First — Prepare for an easier fast by a gradually changing diet toward a mucusless diet, and natural herbal laxatives and enemas.

Second — Change shorter fasts periodically with some eating days of cleansing "mucus-poor" and mucusless diet.

Third — Be particularly careful if the patient used much drugs; especially if a mercury or salpetre, oxide of silver (taken for venereal diseases) have been used, in which case a long, slowly changing, preparative diet is advisable.

An "expert's" suggestion to fast until the tongue is clean caused many troubles with "fanatical" fasters, and I personally know of one death. You may be surprised when I tell you that I had to cure patients from the ill-effects of too long a fast. The reason will be clear later.

In spite of the above, every cure, and especially every cure of diet should start with a two or three-day fast. Every patient can do this without any harm, regardless of how seriously sick he may be. First a laxative and then an enema daily, makes it easier as well as harmless.

HOW TO BREAK A FAST

I consider the knowledge of how to break a fast of the utmost importance.

The right food after a fast itself. At the same time, it depends entirely upon the condition of the patient, and very much upon the length of the fast. You may learn from the results of the two extreme cases, both of which ended fatally — not from the fast, but from the first wrong meal — just why this knowledge is so important.

A one-sided meat eater, suffering from diabetes, broke his fast which lasted about a week by eating dates and died from the effects. A man of over 60 years of age fasted twenty-eight days (too long); his first meal of vegetarian foods consisting mainly of boiled potatoes. A necesary operation showed that the potatoes were kept in the contracted intestines by thick, sticky mucus so strong that a piece had to be cut off and the patient died shortly after the operation.

In the first case the terrible poisons loosened in the stomach of this one-sided meat eater during his fast when mixed with the concentrated fruit sugar of the dates, caused at once so great a fermentation with carbonic acid gases and other poisons that the patient could not stand the shock. The correct advice would be: First a laxative, such as a preparation consisting of harmless herbs, later raw and cooked starchless vegetables, a piece of rough bran bread toast. Sauerkraut is to be recommended in such cases. No fruits should be eaten for a long time after the fast has been broken. The patient should have been prepared for the fast by a longer transition diet.

In the second case the patient fasted entirely too long for a man of his age without proper preparation.

Thru these two very instructive examples you may see how individually different the advice must be, and how wrong it is to make up general suggestions concerning how to break a fast.

Important Rules for the Faster

TO BE CAREFULLY STUDIED AND MEMORIZED

What can be said in general, and what I teach is new and different from the average fasting experts, and is as follows:

1 — The first meal and the menus for a few days after a fast must be of a laxative effect, and not of nourishing value as mostly all others think.

2 — The sooner the first meal passes thru the body the more efficiently it carries out the loosened mucus and poisons of the intestines and the stomach.

3 — If no good stool is experienced after two or three hours — help with laxatives and enemas. Whenever I fasted I always experienced a good bowel movement at least one hour after eating, and at once felt fine. After breaking a long fast I spent more time on the toilet than in bed the following night — and that was as it should be.

While sojourning in Italy many years ago, I drank about two quarts of fresh grape juice after a fast. At once, I experienced a watery diarrhea set in foaming mucus. Almost immediately after I experienced a feeling of such unusual strength that I easily performed the knee-bending and arm-stretching exercise 326 times. This removal so thoroughly of obstructions, taking place after a fast of a few days, increased "P" — vitality at once! You will have to experience a similar sensation to believe me, and then you will agree with my formula, "Vitality equals Power minus Obstructions," and you will realize the absurdity of making up scientific nourishing menus for health and efficiency.

4 — The longer the fast the more efficiently the bowels perform after it is over.

5 — The best laxative foods after a fast are fresh sweet fruits; best of all are cherries and grapes, then a little soaked or stewed prunes. These fruits **must not be used after a meateater's first fast,** but only for people who have lived for a certain time on mucusless or at least mucus-poor foods — the "transition diet."

6 — In the average case it is advisable to break the fast with raw and cooked starchless vegetables; stewed spinach has an especially good effect.

7 — If the first meal does not cause any unpleasantness, you may eat as much as you can. Eating only a small quantity of food for the first 2 or 3 days without experiencing a bowel movement — owing to the small amount of food taken — (another wrong advice given by "experts") — is dangerous.

8 — If you are in the proper condition so that you can start eating with fruits, and you have no bowel movement after about an hour, then eat more or eat a vegetable meal as suggested above, eat until you bring out the waste accumulated during the fast with your stool, after eating the first meal.

Rules During the Fast

1 — Clean the lower intestines as well as you can with enemas, at least every other day.

2 — Before starting a longer fast, take a laxative occasionally, and by all means the day before you start the fast.

3 — If possible, remain in the fresh air, day and night.

4 — Take a walk, exercise, or some other physical work only when you feel strong enough to do it; if tired and weak, rest and sleep as much as you can.

5 — On days when you feel weak, and you will experience such days when the waste is in the circulation, you will find that your sleep is restless and disturbed, and you may

experience bad dreams. This is caused thru the poisons passing thru the brain. Doubt — loss of faith, will arise in your mind; then take this lesson and read it over and over, as well as the other fasting chapters, and especially Lesson 5 of my Mucusless Diet Healing System book. Don't forget that you are, parenthetically speaking, lying on Nature's operating table; the most wonderful of all operations that could be performed; and without the use of a knife! If any extraordinary sensation occurs due to the drugs that are now in circulation, **take an enema at once, lie down, and if necessary break the fast, but not with fruits.**

6 — Whenever you arise after lying down, do it slowly; otherwise you may become dizzy. The latter condition is not serious, but you had better avoid it in this manner. It caused me a considerable fear in the beginning, and I know a number of fasters and strict eaters who gave up when they experienced this sensation — lost their faith forever.

FASTING DRINKS

The "fanatic" fasting enthusiast drinks only water. He thinks it best to avoid any trace of food whatever. I CONSIDER A LIGHT LEMONADE WITH A LITTLE HONEY OR BROWN SUGAR OR A LITTLE FRUIT JUICE THE BEST. Drink as often as you care to during the day, but in general, not more than 2 to 3 quarts a day. The less you drink the more aggressive the fast works.

As a change, vegetable juice made from cooked starchless vegetables is very good during a longer fast. Raw tomato juice, etc., is also good. But if fruit juice, for example, orange juice, is used during a longer fast, be extremely careful because the fruit juices may cause the poisons to become loosened too rapidly without causing a bowel movement. I know a number of such fruit and fruit-juice fasts which failed completely because all mucus and all poisons loosened too fast and too much at one time, disturbs all organs too greatly when in the circulation, and have to be eliminated only thru the circulation without the aid of bowel movements.

MORNING FAST OR NON-BREAKFAST PLAN

The worst of all eating habits nowadays is to stuff the stomach with food early in the morning. In European countries, excepting England, no one takes a regular meal for breakfast; it is generally a drink of some kind with bread only.

The only time that man does not eat for 10 or 12 hours is while he is asleep during the night. As soon as his stomach is free from food, the body starts the eliminating process of a fast; therefore encumbered people feel miserable and have a coated tongue upon awakening in the morning. They have no appetite at all, yet they crave food, eat it, and feel better — WHY?

ANOTHER MYSTERY REVEALED

This is one of the greatest problems I solved, and is one that has puzzled all "experts" who believe it is the food itself. As soon as you refill the stomach with food, THE ELIMINATION IS STOPPED and you feel better! I must say that this secret which I discovered is undoubtedly the explanation of why eating became a habit and is no longer what nature intended it should be, i.e., a satisfaction, a compensation of nature's need of food.

This habit of eating, striking all civilized mankind and now physiologically explained, involves and proves the saying I coined long ago — "Life is a tragedy of nutrition." The more waste that man accumulates, the more he must eat to stop the elimination. I had patients who had to eat several times during the night to be able to sleep again. In other words, they had to put food in the stomach to avoid the digestion of mucus and poisons, accumulated there.

Short Fasts and the Non-Breakfast Plan

During my experience with thousands of fasters I had patients that had to eat several times during the night in order to sleep again. The reason is very apparent. Let me cite an example. Upon awakening you perhaps feel fine — but instead of getting up you remain in bed and fall asleep again — have a bad dream, and actually feel miserable upon awakening the second time. You can understand the exact reason for this.

As soon as you get up, walk around or do something the body is in an entirely different condition than during the sleep. The elimination is slowed down, the energy being used elsewhere.

If eating breakfast is eliminated from your daily menus, you will probably experience some harmless sensation, such as headaches for the first one or two days, but after that you will feel much better, work better, and enjoy your luncheon better than ever. Hundreds of severe cases have been cured by the "non-breakfast-Fast" alone, without important changes in diet; proving that the habit of a full breakfast meal is the worst of all, and most injurious.

It is advisable and really of great advantage to allow the patient to have the same drink for breakfast that he is accustomed to; if he craves coffee, let him continue his drink of coffee, but absolutely no SOLID food! Later on, replace the coffee with a warm vegetable juice, and still later change to lemonade. This change should be made gradually for the average mixed eater.

THE 24-HOUR FAST, OR ONE MEAL A DAY PLAN

As with the breakfast-fast you can heal more severe cases with the 24-hour fast, for in cases of deep chronic encumbrance and drugs it is a careful, preliminary step to the necessary longer fasts. The best time to eat is in the afternoon, say, 3 or 4 o'clock P.M.

If the patient is on the mucusless or transition diet, let him eat the fruits first — (fruits should always be eaten first) — and after an elapse of 15 or 20 minutes eat the vegetables; but all should be eaten within an hour so that it is to say, one meal.

FASTING WHEN USED IN CONNECTION WITH THE MUCUSLESS DIET HEALING SYSTEM

As I have stated before, I am no longer in favor of long fasts. In fact it may become criminal to let a patient fast for 30 or 40 days on water — contracting the avenues of circulation — which are continually filling up more and more with mucus, and by dangerous old drugs and poisons, and at the same time rotten blood from his old "stock" — in fact, actually starving from necessary vital food elements. No one can stand a fast of that kind without disadvantage or without harming his vitality.

If fasting is to be used at all, then start at first with the non-breakfast plan; then follow with the 24-hour fast for a while; then gradually increase up to 3, 4 or 5-day fasts, eating between fasts for 1, 2, 3 or 4 days a mucusless diet, combined individually as an elimination adjustment, and at the same time supplying and rebuilding the body continually with and by the best elements contained in and found only in mucusless foods.

Thru such intermittent fasts the blood is gradually improved, regenerated, can more easily tolerate the poisons and waste, and the patient is able at the same time to dissolve and eliminate "disease deposits" from the deepest tissues of the body; deposits that no doctor ever dreamed existed, and that no other method of healing has ever discovered or can remove.

This, then, is the Mucusless Diet Healing System, with fasting an essential part of it.

FASTING IN CASES OF ACUTE DISEASE

"Hunger Cures — Wonder Cures" was the title of the first fasting book I ever read. It gave the experiences of a country doctor, in which he said, "No feverish, acute disease, must nor can end with death if nature's instinctive command, to stop eating thru lack of appetite, is followed."

It is insanity to give food to a pneumonia patient with a high fever, for instance. Having had an unusual contraction of the lung tissues by a "cold" the pressed-out mucus goes into the circulation and produces an unusual heat-fever. The human engine, already thru heat, at the bursting point, becomes more heated thru partaking of solid food, meat broth, etc. (good nourishing foods).

Air-baths taken in the room, enemas, laxatives, cool lemon-ade would save the lives of thousands of young men who are now daily permitted to die, the innocent victims of pneumonia, or other acute diseases — due to the stubborn ignorance of doctors and so-called highly civilized people.

Fasting for Spiritual Rebirth Thru the Superior Fast

All experts, except myself, believe that you live from your own flesh during a fast. You know now, that what they call metabolism — "metabolize your own flesh when you fast" is simply the elimination of waste.

The Indian "fakir," the greatest fakir in the world today, is nothing but skin and bones. I learned that the cleaner you are, the easier it is to fast, and the longer you can stand it. In other words: In a body free from all waste and poisons, and when no solid foods are taken, the human body functions for the first time in its life without obstructions. The elasticity of the entire tissue system, and of the internal organs, especially of the spongy lungs, work with an entirely different vibration and efficiency than ever before, by air alone and without the slightest obstructions. Stated differently: "V" equals "P" and if you simply supply the "engine" with the necessary water which is used up, you ascend into a higher state of physical, mental and spiritual condition. I call that the "Superior fast."

If your blood "stock" is formed from eating the foods I teach, your brain will function in a manner that will surprise you. Your former life will take on the appearance of a dream, and for the first time in your existence your conscience awakens to a real self-consciousness.

Your mind, your thinking, your ideals, your aspirations and your philosophy change fundamentally in such a way as to beggar description.

Your soul will shout for joy and triumph over all misery of life leaving it all behind you. For the first time, you will feel a vibration of vitality thru your body — like a slight electric current — that shakens you delightfully.

You will learn and realize that fasting and superior fasting (and not volumes of psychology and philosophy) is the real and only key to a superior life; to the revelation of a superior world, and to the spiritual world.

All of my "experiments" were made on my own person, before being used on patients. My health experiments began while still holding a professorship in Baden-Baden, Germany, where I had become "incurably ill". My complete restoration to health — to what was probably the most perfect state of health of anyone living in our Western civilization today, was an interesting adventure of finding the fundamental laws of nature during my pursuit of health. I found that the body normalizes itself if properly cleansed of toxic wastes and supplied with proper nutrition. "MUCUS" is the key-note of the misunderstanding. I have consistently and definitely proven that a "mucusless diet" —coupled with the wise use of Fasting, and observing the basic laws of physiology, is the "magic wand" by which our present day civilization will be afforded a new lease on life. I contend that all disease, regardless of its "scientific" name, or the symptoms accompanying it — consists of constitutional encumbrance of waste material known as "foreign matter." Nature continually attempts to eliminate this disease producing waste encumbrance and to stop the source of it. My method of restoration performs exactly the same in the human body as instinctive self-healing does in the animal kingdom. The disease producing material is partially digested, decaying, semi-liquid generally known as "mucus". Everyone living on todays, accepted mixed diet consisting of starchy vegetables, grains and meat is more or less clogged up with "mucus", — whether sick or not!

Conclusion

While I have conducted thousands of Fasting cures, any number of people have been helped by simply changing their present dietary habits. The sudden change of diet causes disturbances even in an entirely healthy person. For this reason a change made too rapidly may become dangerous and a complete knowledge is therefore essential.

To relieve and avoid any disturbance of health and at the same time to replace the old "tid-bit" enjoyments by new and better ones can be accomplished if one follows my transition diet. Changing from meat eating to a strictly vegetarian or fruitarian diet always results in a more vigorous feeling for the first few days; then weakness, great fatigue, possibly headaches and palpitation of the heart set in.

Fruit being the only natural food, loosens and dissolves the mucus, poisons and toxemias and the penned up filth and morass of over-feeding is passed out thru the circulating blood. The dead, decayed tissues are pushed aside to make room for the new living food substances and for the time being the patient loses the change of matter balance. The elimination of poison thru the circulating blood causes more or less disturbance of health. And unless you are thoroughly convinced of the efficacy of the natural diet your friends will dissuade you from further attempts to cleanse the body and will urge an interruption of internal purification in order to save you from what they believe will result seriously and you will soon become lean, the face will appear haggard and drawn and a general depression of feeling may overtake you. This, then, is the healing crisis and if understandingly carried on will result in unhoped for good health. I divide all foods into two kinds.

1. Mucus-forming foods.
2. Non-mucus-forming foods.

Under the first heading we find meat, eggs, fats, milk and all by-products made therefrom, dried beans, dried peas, lentils and ALL STARCHY FOODS.

The second classification embraces: All non-starchy green vegetables and all kinds of fruits. There are certain vegetables and fruits that contain more or less starch and should be given the place of secondary importance in the dietary.

Begin the transition with as much mucus-less foods as possible and as little mucus-forming foods as possible. I call this a mucus-less diet. The next step towards health is the MUCUS-LESS DIET, which means a combination of starchless vegetables and fruits. With the help of this transition diet and some knowledge by the individual to choose and combine rightly, the greatest and most important truth of life is revealed to him. The mis-called strength which we experience after meat-eating is nothing but stimulation, for there is no nourishment for man in meat. Hardening of the arteries, in which fatty, plaque-shaped particles are deposited on the blood vessel walls. They build up a choking lining; in time they may calcify and harden. High-blood pressure often results. This kind of hardening of the arteries is the chief villain in death and disability. Heart attacks, arthritis and diseases of senilty stem from this same cause. The meat-eating animals will die on cooked meats without blood and bones! And rats soon die on an exclusive diet of white flour.

My mucus theory — now a proven fact — has been more and more recognized. It has withstood the test with enormous success and today has a platform that: NATURAL TREATMENT AND DIET IS THE MOST PERFECT AND SUCCESSFUL SYSTEM OF HEALING KNOWN.

Nothing is easier than making promises merely by saying words — and nothing is more difficult than actually living up to these easily made promises day after day! What you promise today must be renewed and re-decided tomorrow. For you and no one else but you, must decide the "want to live." Ehret's health teachings; based on a natural diet over the years that lie ahead must be followed. You will soon find life more desirable, and you will enter with joyous gusto into things you formerly feared! A whole new vista will be opened to you!

Suffering humanity may now have the means of not only relieving but PREVENTING disease, thru Rational Fasting and the Mucusless Diet and developing an improved race of people that need never know what diseased conditions are. And my most fervent hope is that it will bring about a better civilized humanity.

May this book serve all readers seeking after truth regardless of its source; may it especially serve the sick and encourage those worrying about the loss of their youth, and the first sign of old age. And may this book find an increasingly larger audience who will accept and follow the truths it teaches — for fasting is not a fad but a definite cure which must eventually establish itself in a permanent first place to the benefit of all mankind.

—END—

Health and Happiness Through Fasting

WHEN – WHY – WHERE AND HOW TO FAST.

by

Fred S. Hirsch

Health and Happiness Through Fasting
When - Why - Where and How - To Fast

by
Fred S. Hirsch

FASTING requires much more knowledge than the average health seeker considers necessary. Hopefully, this article will help convince you that through fasting lies the road to health and happiness. Few individuals pay much attention to the underlying causes of human illness, or the vital problems of what food is best for human consumption, and as a result we innocently contribute to our own miseries and ailments through over-indulgence in eating incompatible food combinations; i.e., meat, alcoholic stimulants, dairy products and starchy foods, excessive worry, tension and over-work are all contributing factors.

FASTING must first be recognized as Nature's way of healing all ills, and while not a "cure-all" for every known ailment, total fasting makes it possible for Nature in her desperate and continuous effort; to remove and expel the foreign matter and disease producing toxemic wastes from the body thereby correcting the faults of wrong living and improper diet.

FASTING may not be adapted to everyone, under every condition, but fortunately, fasting can prove acceptable to the great majority. Nature alone possesses the true healing power and our body can therefore be designated a "self-curative" organism. For centuries past we have been taught to look upon illness, "disease", as some deliberate affliction visited upon us whether deserved or not — whereas in truth it is actually Nature's "house-cleaning" effort! When this truism finally becomes recognized, and Nature, the great healer is permitted to carry on, you will note a vast improvement in your health. Suppressing ailments and symptoms of pain through use of sedative and pain relieving drugs must eventually result in the illness becoming chronic. During the course of a life time toxemic wastes are continually being discharged and it is claimed that the body and all vital organs have been renewed many times. Correcting wrong dietetic habits will permit the body to take advantage of this natural phenomenon and build clean healthy tissue! **Only through a total fast can this be satisfactorily brought about.** Voluntary abstinence from food for restoring normal bodily vigor was instinctive with primitive man. Start fasting one or two days, drinking water only, to which a few drops of lemon or lime juice has been added, especially if distilled water is used. At about four or five o'clock in the afternoon, break the fast with a light laxative or enema. You will be shocked at the amount of waste that is now being thrown off almost immediately. This mass of previously uneliminated waste was poisoning your blood stream circulation continuously. This should help convince you that here is the way — and the only way, to health!

It is the height of folly to expect modern "miracle drugs" to do more than to temporarily suppress the aches and pains of "disease". Because of the sedative ability of the narcotic drug to deaden the inflamed nerves and tissues for a few hours at most, Nature's "warning signals" are thereby ruthlessly disregarded! Arnold Ehret truthfully claims that "the basic cause of all latent disease of man, whatever its official name may be, is a clogged up tissue system of uneliminated, unused and undigested food substances. Disease is still a mystery to every Doctor who fails, or deliberately refuses, to understand and recognize these simple facts!" Disease consists of a "foreign matter" which has weight, and which must be eliminated from the body before the patient can hope to get well. Every sick person must, therefore, go through the healing process of a "cleansing" so that the body may have the opportunity of eliminating the sticky "mucus", which has been stored in the tissues or held in the pockets of the intestines for years and which interfere with the proper digestive and blood-building functions. Unfortunately, fasting is so feared by the average individual that he actually believes starvation will result thru missing a few meals — when in reality he is being helped, and many practitioners fail to grasp, or fully understand, that there is a vast difference existing between fasting and starvation. A sure proof of the efficacy of fasting is to discontinue all food intake, with the exception of water, for a day or two. Note how the tongue (being an organ of elimination) becomes thickly coated with mucus. The odor of decaying foods is on your breath and the bowel eliminations become offensive. Probably for the first time the body has now been given an opportunity of eliminating the over-abundance of stored up wastes and encumbrances clogging up the tissues! Having assured yourself of the desirability of ridding your body of unwanted waste and encumbrances, the remedy consists of a series of short fasts — each fast to be followed by a "cleansing diet" of fruits and green leaf vegetables, eaten either in their natural or cooked state. This "cleansing program" must be continued just so long as complete recovery to normal health is absent.

How Long Should One Fast

Every person has an individual problem — age of patient, nature of the illness, amount and type of drugs previously used. In fact, so many considerations need be given full recognition of this subject that the list would be endless. Fasting is Nature's oldest, yet least expensive, and in our opinion, best method of treating disease. In fact, fasting can be considered the cornerstone of Natural Healing, and its value without equal. How long should one fast becomes important since long fasts of thirty to fifty days could become dangerous unless properly conducted and supervised by a knowledgeable authority. It is therefore wisest, for the faster to adopt a series of short fasts, i.e.: two or three days of each week, gradually increasing the length of each succeeding fast, a day or more if necessary, but not to exceed more than a week of total fast at one time. This will enable the chronically ill body to gradually and slowly eliminate these toxic waste materials responsible for their illness without seriously affecting normal body functioning, after which a corrected mode of living will restore the individual to a virile, vigorous state of health. Fasting for overcoming both acute and chronic ailments is centuries old — dating back to the beginning of life itself. No claim is made that fasting is necessarily a pleasant experience, yet the faster often receives blessed relief from physical pain, plus self-satisfaction, in the knowledge that the fast might eventually result in complete cessation of all pain and, hopefully, a return to normalcy! Primarily, a fast is undertaken for a good reason — the individual is desirous of correcting and overcoming illness, or a depleted loss of vital power which has already manifested itself threatens to become chronic — so the answer to "how long should one fast", becomes clear — i.e.: continue the short fasts until the illness has been overcome and disease no longer exists! This suggestion, of course, refers directly to the length of time that the series of "shorter fasts", as previously outlined, are to be continued.

Why to Fast

The search for health goes on unceasingly and while fasting has helped untold thousands of sufferers to regain normal health it is essential that we must know when, how and why to fast in order that we might receive the greater amount of physical and mental benefit.

Arnold Ehret in his "Mucusless Diet Healing System" tells us: "Every disease, no matter what name it may be known by in medical science, is CONSTIPATION, i.e., — a clogging up of the entire pipe system of the human body." Please note that Ehret uses the word "constipation" to apply to "a clogging up (a constipation) of the entire human pipe system" and not merely a "bowel evacuation", the ordinarily accepted usage of the word. He refers specifically to the accumulation of waste toxic matters in the tissues and in the blood stream, the lungs, kidneys, bladder, stomach, intestinal tract — in fact, every organ of the entire body. And since in Ehret's opinion 99-9/10% of all ailments directly result from the same causes, he aptly refers to all common ailments as "the oneness of disease." Hence, the method of correction of the common cold, bronchitis, asthma, sinusitis or tuberculosis, can best be accomplished through fasting since in his opinion all ailments are the direct result of a "clogged up" overloaded mucus condition brought about through wrong dietetic habits — i.e.: the over-eating of "mucus-forming" types of food.

The simple remedial expedient is to discontinue doing that which was the original cause of the condition. Fast, and thereby give Nature an opportunity to eliminate these "toxic waste matters" which Ehret calls "mucus". High blood pressure, migraine or other types of headches, cardiac conditions or peptic ulcers, colitis, rickets, anemia, neuritis or acidosis, epilepsy, glaucoma, urinary disturbances of the bladder, nephritis, tumors, or even sterility, to name but just a few, according to Ehret's teachings, consists of an overloaded mucus condition existing throughout the entire body, directly traceable to the one great dietic sin — gluttonous over-eating of incorrect food mixtures. Ehret's claim that 99-9/10% of all ailments actually result from the one cause, wrong food combinations and "gluttony"; remains unshaken! Forcing ourselves to eat when no appetite exists because of the prevalent and popular belief that we must eat to gain strength and vitality, can result in the temporary loss of all desire for food of any kind and, unfortunately, the results of this forced eating of — "plenty of good nourishing foods" may actually produce an entirely opposite result! We end up building disease rather than gaining vitality — and ofttimes permanent illness is the net result! All of which teaches us that strength, vitality and good health are by no means dependent upon the *quantity* of our food intake but rather through the actual amount of properly digested and assimilated food eaten that can be used by the body.

Fasting can start you on the road to the fulfillment of an enjoyable, pleasant, happy way of life; and the end result of following a natural method of eating and living is a longer, healthful life! These are but a few "why to fast" reasons.

When and How to Fast

Dr. Frank McCoy, in his book, "The Fast Way to Health", recounts hundreds of cases who were greatly helped through an exclusive liquid diet consisting of nothing but fresh orange juice. The patient reported to Dr. McCoy's office daily, for periods of from three to six weeks. Besides the orange juice diet other modalities, such as massage, vibrating machines, colonic irrigations and Chiropractic adjustments, were also used in the treatment to help keep the patient occupied, but Dr. McCoy gives full credit to the fast. Bernarr McFadden, the well-known Physical Culturist, received much publicity through advocating an exclusive milk diet and thousands of persons claim to have received great benefit from this diet. Both modalities the fresh orange juice, and milk diet, come under the category of what could be called a "camouflaged fast." In other words, the body is permitted to "rest" and rebuild since the one type of food only, requires considerably less vitality to digest. The over-worked organs are thus given an opportunity to slow down, thereby strengthening the patient's vitality. Unused morbid waste encumbrances are eliminated and the previously overworked body can now carry on the normal digestive process. An exclusive "milk diet" can cause constipation and for this reason has proven undesirable. The fresh orange juice diet, if used by a patient heavily encumbered with concentrated poisons, could cause these concentrated poisons to be released into the blood stream, too rapidly and in fact it might even be conceivable, without proper supervision this condition could end disastrously.

To attempt a long fast, and at the same time continue to carry on our daily chores or work as usual, is not entirely fair to the faster since, after all, we must not overlook the fact that during the fast we are actually on "Nature's operating table". A considerable amount of bodily vitality is consumed during the process of throwing off these age-old "poisons and toxic waste materials", and justifiably a complete rest — even to the point of remaining in bed during the entire period of the fast, is often indicated. In other words, a complete physical rest and mental relaxation should be the rule if at all possible during such strenuous "housecleansing" periods. The form of fasting known as a liquid diet, especially if the liquid consist of fresh fruit or vegetable juices or cooked vegetable broth (celery, carrots, parsley, onions, tomatoes, etc.) can be continued a month or more without overtaxing the patient's vital forces. But when fresh grapes, orange or grapefruit juice is used exclusively considerably more caution must be the rule since these particular juices bring extremely aggressive, have a decidedly potent ability to "stir-up" toxic wastes. Thrown into the blood circulation too rapidly, especially after a long total fast when the eliminated poisons are in concentrated form, the blood stream becomes "overloaded" and normal body functioning is seriously disarranged. Dizzy spells might occur, followed by severe diarrhea and vomiting—and while this could be only temporary it should require careful observation and attention. In case this physical reaction persists it is advisable, and imperative, to discontinue the fast immediately, and a diet of cooked vegetables containing much roughage, such as celery, carrots, cabbage, squash, spinach, beets, sauerkraut, etc., or even meats (particularly if the patient has been a one-sided meat eater) temporarily, at least until the body functioning returns to normal and all symptoms of dizziness have completely disappeared. When cooked or all baked types of fruits and vegetables, including the fresh frozen fruits and vegetables, are much less "aggressive" as far as their eliminating ability is concerned. Now you may appreciate why it is so necessary that you take into consideration the amount of existing waste and "poisonous" toxic matters in your body before undertaking a long fast. Even the innocent appearing "soothing syrups" given to infants contain some form of "narcotics" in minute dosage — hence, the extreme importance of having complete knowledge before suggesting a long fast is so essential in more ways than one.

We need only to look to the animal world to learn the importance that wise Mother Nature places in fasting. All sick, seriously ill, or wounded animals immediately discontinue eating food and go on a total fast in a secluded place where they can relax from all activity until they have completely regained their health and vigor. This could require a period of time as long as a week or even a month, but their patience is always rewarded with success. Complete fasting without food or water of a number of animals during their long winter hibernation is a well known phenomenon, and it is even customary for many animals to fast during the "nursing period", remaining with their young until weaned. Fasting must be recognized as a natural and safe method of care of the sick body, a method by which the person is enabled to overcome illness through eliminating, almost miraculously, the cause of the ailment, and yet it can be said there is nothing "miraculous" about it! Whether we fast to restore health, gain or lose weight, or merely to retain our present bodily vigor, we soon recognize that fasting is a vital factor through which we may increase our vitality and personal well-being, both mentally and physically. Besides readily overcoming such minor discomforts as the common cold or indigestion, fasting, undoubtedly, adds to your life span! The digestive process uses up precious vitality — contrariwise, fasting has been known to actually rebuild vital forces, and the conclusion must become self-evident that fasting prolongs life itself! It is necessary, therefore, that we repeat over and over again the importance of entering upon a fast intelligently, confident in the final outcome, with complete understanding and knowledge, and we specifically refer to the longer fasts. It is essential, for example, that the faster knows the difference between "false" and "real" appetite. Hunger pains caused through "false appetite" can generate rather severe pains in the stomach region, together with various emotional disturbances and a corresponding feeling of weakness. Since the eating of food will at this period immediately cause stoppage of the distress symptoms it is only natural for the faster to surmise that lack of food was the cause, and eating; the remedy, whereas the opposite might be true. Our established life-long habit of eating "by the clock" has firmly affixed in our minds the desirability of eating at that precise time. The fact of the matter is that true hunger can only take place when a real need for food exists! The individual who is always hungry is, in fact, "pathologically unwell". Surely no need for food exists when hunger is lacking. Never force yourself to eat unless you are *truly* hungry and a keen relish for food exists. Otherwise, you merely add work to an already "overworked" digestive tract. All excess food becomes a burden and this, of course, is especially true in case of illness. Over-eating, or forced feeding, retards recovery by requiring the body to use its precious vitality in the elimination of this un-needed food. Often this so called "good nourishing" diet is actually to blame for the patient's loss of weight and lessened vitality! Even in the healthy body, when over-eating or gluttony is indulged in, it can cause vomiting and diarrhea, for the healthy organ rejects all excess food. Contrariwise, when the quantity of food intake is decreased (lessened) bodily energy is conserved since the digestive organs have less work to do — liver, pancreas, heart and arteries are relieved of a greater portion of their labor, all of which, naturally, results in an increase of the healing process! Witholding all food intake from the sick patient causes every depurating organ in the entire body to increase its eliminating activity, It starts immediately to get rid of all poisonous wastes and a cleansing of the entire tissue system begins. Nothing equals the fast as a means of eliminating age-old stored up wastes from an over-loaded tissue system. Nature's constant and unceasing effort, therefore, is to remove all unusable and excess waste substances from the body and fortunately for us this constant elimination goes on continuously and good health is the result. To be willing to settle for half health, or less, when real health is possible is to rob yourself of life's most precious possession. Aristotle, that great Greek philosopher, said over 2300 years ago — "If there is one way better than another, it is the way of Nature". Much vital energy is required during this cleansing process, but paradoxical as it might seem, the faster usually gains both in strength and weight. The feverish patient already lacks the necessary vitality to digest food while suffering pain yet "nourishing food" continues to be advised. Unfortunately, the popular idea that man must eat every few hours in order to stay alive remains; despite the fact that it has been proven over and over again that the "sick person" actually gains in strength when food is withheld and suffers a relapse from forced feeding! How many thousands of patients have been innocently "fed" into premature graves through ignorance of Nature's laws? No claim is herein made that fasting alone, regardless of the advanced stage of the illness, or bodily and mental condition of the patient will produce the sure cure. Common sense and caution must be your guide during the fast and we can safely predict that in the majority of cases the faster will become physically stronger and more vital and mentally alert — up to the point, of course, that the individual is capable of accepting. Unfortunately, fasting, when used in far advanced cases as a last resort, or in long standing chronic cases, especially in the elderly person of lowered vitality, cannot be expected to produce the "miracle". Terminal cases, for example, can only hope for a lessening of the discomfort of their pain. Total fasting is not indicated in these terminal cases but worthwhile results, merely through reducing the quantity of food intake, are often experienced. An extremely limited, carefully selected diet, in all cases should be carried on — and, remember, over-feeding can only result in increased suffering. Dr. J. H. Tilden, M.D., conducted thousands of fasts in his Denver Sanitarium and authored many books on the subject of fasting. He wrote, "I must say in all seriousness that fasting when combined with a properly selected diet is the nearest approach to a 'cure-all' that is possible to conceive — profoundly simple and simply profound!"

Without exception, all of the modern "miracle drugs", including Aspirin drugs employed today to restore the sick and ailing to normal health, have been known to result in great bodily harm. It is well known, and readily acknowledged, that they act as a palliative and not a cure, yet often the ill effects they cause are not discovered until many years after taking, before reactions occur in the affected organ and are recognized. When the cause of illness is finally removed and the restorative process of true healing is given the opportunity to function Nature's remarkable "rebuilding" process takes place and proceeds in an orderly manner in accordance with Natural Physiological Law! Wounds are healed, broken bones are mended, destroyed tissues are replaced, and we can positively state that these healing processes have never been duplicated through any method or laboratory finding as yet devised by mere man! It is true that the scientist has kept living tissue alive and growing in his laboratory, but he has never been able to reproduce living tissue, nor has he developed a man-made substitute for the natural life process through which healing is accomplished! Nature's healing process starts instantly when the need occurs, and we must recognize the importance of aiding Nature through fasting, since we now know that the healing process increases when the body is freed from disposing of surplus food. Only a total abstinence from food makes it possible for the sick body to function thoroughly, in its own inimitable way, during the healing period. As previously mentioned, Arnold Ehret preferred the so-called "short fast" of three days to a week or ten days for the average individual. It was his experience that satisfactory results could be obtained through a series of so-called "shorter" fasts, especially in cases where the patient is not under competent supervision and "on his own" so to speak. It is well for the individual to decide on how long he intends to carry on before initiating the fast. Let us say, for example, that the patient is of the "nervous", high-strung or imaginative type, or he may even be skeptical of results that might occur. He must first of all create an enthusiastic desire to fast. If the slightest doubt of final success is permitted to enter his mind then not more than two or three days should be the extent of the fast in this case. Hopefully, the resulting good feeling will quiet all future unnecessary fears, and the next fast can be for a longer period, even up to a full week.

The over-weight individual finds it much easier to go without food. Loss of weight causes no fear, and the patient's mental attitude makes fasting almost a pleasure! A week, or perhaps ten days for this type of individual, brings practically no discomfort whatsoever. The first day's hunger pangs perhaps are the most difficult. A mouthful of water (held for ten or fifteen minutes before expectorating) will lessen the "false appetite" craving for food, which decreases as the fast progresses. The seriously sick, or severely injured individual, has absolutely no desire for food, so fasting comes naturally. A safe rule to follow is to stop eating until appetite has returned, or until you feel completely well.

When to Fast

Nature has selected the spring of the year for the annual "house-cleansing" period. The very types of the first green leaf vegetables and fruits that Nature brings forth and amply supplies in the early spring give significant testimony to this fact. The green leaf vegetables and herbs are proven blood purifiers, well known over the centuries, and because of their laxative qualities they are recognized efficient "cleansers".

This same description applies as well to the first fruits of the season. Cherries, for example, one of the earlier fruits to ripen, have long been recognized for their "cleansing" ability. Their enticing color appeal, plus the sweet and delicious flavor, particularly when gathered and eaten direct from the tree, will produce remarkable blood purifying and "cleansing" results. An exclusive cherry diet for five or six days is a "camouflaged fast" well worth trying. Since the body's resistance to cold weather is lowered during the fast it is more pleasant to fast during the warmer weather, but this is not to say that we should wait until warm weather returns before undertaking a fast if the need for fasting exists. Postponing the fast, awaiting warmer weather could prove inadvisable for a delay might conceivably result in the ailment becoming more involved. It is very easy for the patient to remain indoors while fasting and remain comfortable during the coldest weather.

Why to Fast

Fasting is indicated in many instances. At the first indication of the "common cold" for example, fasting becomes a preventative measure! Start the "cleansing" (fasting) program before a more serious, chronic condition develops! Minor ailments such as headaches, biliousness, nervousness, injuries and even excessive grief, all indicate the desirability of missing a meal or two. The length of time must, of course, depend entirely on the condition of the faster. For more serious ailments, the amount of toxic waste and foreign encumbrances present in the blood stream must be taken into consideration and often a longer fast is indicated. Age of the faster is another important factor since we cannot expect to overcome the effects of a life time of wrong living within a few short days, or weeks. The chronic sufferer, therefore, must exercise patience and perseverance in his efforts to return to normal health. It is to be expected that in many instances the faster becomes discouraged, even frightened, at the actual results that the fast brings about during the early stages of the "house-cleansing" period. But with complete faith and knowledge of what is actually occurring the final results will eventually prove very worthwhile. A little "self-discipline" would provide many of us with a steady flow of energy and a wonderful sense of inner well being that comes from a healthy body.

Where to Fast

Often times where to fast must be given a great deal of consideration. The inevitable opposition of the well-meaning members of the "family" often proves to be the most difficult of the obstacles to overcome. Our loved ones, because of the inborn fear of starvation inculcated in all of us since early childhood, find it impossible to withhold well intentioned warnings and often plead tearfully with the faster to "eat something". They honestly and sincerely believe that great bodily harm, even death itself, will inevitably result from a fast of more than a few days at most! Their pleadings when ignored often lead to hysterical and angry efforts to force the faster to "eat some good nourishing food" and the unfortunate sick person, already weakened through illness, loses his original determination to "get well or else" — and succumbs to their pleadings by "eating something" which often are the very foods that should not be used! It may well be that the faster himself is not completely "sold" to the efficacy of the fast — in which case he can be more easily swayed from his original plan to continue the fast, since he lacks the courage of his own convictions. Should this experience be yours, then at least eat the foods that you know are indicated for breaking the fast, as taught by Prof. Arnold Ehret, in order to accomplish the most good. It might be wise under these conditions to arrange for suitable supervision at a sanitarium or rest home specializing in fasting, particularly if the faster contemplates a longer fast of two or three weeks duration. Never lose sight of the fact that the faster is on "Nature's 'bloodless' operating table" and should, therefore, be made comfortable at all times through adequate nursing care, daily sponge baths, massage, colonic irrigations, with complete rest and relaxation, so that the bodily strength and comfort can be retained and even increased. To obey Nature's laws means health—to disregard, whether through ignorance or deliberately, means pain, disease and even death. In other words, health is not merely an accident but an achievement—for the orderly working of the body functions spells HEALTH and its derangement results in disease. The warning signs of pain and discomfort signify that Nature's laws have been digressed, whether unintentionally or not! Freedom from pain, or HEALTH, means that they have been complied with. In the overwhelming majority of illness, all that Nature requires for health to be gained is a discontinuance from doing that which was the original cause of the disease — yet our natural instinct to fast, even missing a single meal, has become lost through present day "civilization" and the increase in all human ills can be directly traced to the accepted customs of our advanced "civilization".

How Long to Fast

The exact length of the fast need not be *definitely* decided beforehand. The various physical and mental reactions which take place during the fast could understandably often cause needless alarm both to the faster and the inexperienced physician. For the first time in years, possibly for the first time in the life of the faster, a thorough cleansing of the tissue system is possible and stored up toxemic wastes and poisons are now being carried off as the avenues of circulation contract permitting the existing over-pressure to be rapidly relieved. Renewed vitality enables the blood stream to discharge the dissolved mucus and toxemic waste materials now in circulation for elimination, and these "poisonous encumbrances" might cause a feeling of being "ill" to exist during this period. You will find, however, that just as soon as the "cleansing process" is completed and the wastes are eliminated, the faster feels stronger than ever before! Ehret often remarked about his fasting patients actually feeling stronger on the third week of the fast than they did during the first week! The unobstructed blood circulation can now produce increased vitality — further proof that Nature heals through fasting. It is this elimination of waste, poisonous materials with which the tissues and intestinal tract have been "clogged up" for years, and now finally removed, that make it possible for normal bodily function to once again take place. It is Nature alone, in the final analysis, through fasting and the resulting elimination of waste materials through the various depurating organs, i.e.: the skin, kidneys, lungs, bowels, as well as our eyes, ears and nose, that aid the true healing process to take place. "The mills of the Gods grind slowly yet they grind exceedingly fine!"

In the final summation we cannot emphasize too strongly the fact that what we know as disease is in reality a "process of purification" — a special effort as it were, on the part of the abused, sick organism to throw off the abnormal quantities of latent poisonous waste materials. Our perverted dietetic habits, the result of false teachings since childhood, are the origin. We attempt to "stop" the pain through unnatural means rather than recognize pain as Nature's warning signal of a local symptom of a general disorder. The majority of persons, never having experienced the feeling of real health and vitality, are not cognizant of what they are missing. They little suspect that mankind's greatest enemies — ignorance, selfishness, greed and gluttony, the cause of all his physical and mental woes exist within himself! Discontinue careless and indulgent over-eating! Comply with Nature's unchangeable laws for safe guidance in your search for health! Fasting gives the body an opportunity to correct these faults of improper dieting — and incompatible food combinations. To enjoy this more abundant, healthier life is within your reach. The sooner you make the decision to start the better off you surely will be. Why not grasp this opportunity and let us help you attain your desired goal of a longer, happier, healthier, more vigorous life.

Become a disciple of health, and prove to yourself that strict, self-discipline brings worthwhile results. Then, thru precept and example, hold high the torch of knowledge and enlightenment to your fellow-man, who while teetering on the very brink of physical and mental collapse finds himself still unable to grasp these simple truths, nor understand the cause of his suffering. Make him anxious to travel the broad road to health leading to a completely new — wonderful, joyous life of physical, spiritual and mental regeneration.

FINIS

ROADS TO
HEALTH AND HAPPINESS

BUILDING STRENGTH
and BODILY EFFICIENCY

INTERNAL CLEANLINESS

MY ROAD TO HEALTH

by
ARNOLD EHRET
and others based on
Ehret's Health Teachings.

CONTENTS

YOUR ROAD TO REGENERATION
Building Bodily Strength and Efficiency
By ARNOLD EHRET

It was during my early thirties that I first became severely sick with Brights disease, and on the very verge of the grave, even after being told by orthodox Medical physicians that my illness was incurable, I fought my way up to an unshaken health that still remains today—a health far better than in the best years of my youth, when I did my military service. I found more or less temporary relief thru different methods of Nature-cure and Drugless healing as practiced at that time, but it became necessary for me to return to nature's infallible remedies—the only methods that can truly overcome disease, and they are: fasting and an exclusive fruit diet!

Neither of these unfailing healing factors were given practically any consideration nor credit for their potential healing abilities by any of the various healing arts of that time. In fact, even today, acknowledgment still continues to be sorely lacking—both by medical science and the average layman who might be interested in his own health regime, but who continues to remain sublimely ignorant. It took years of study, testing and self-experimentation, which often bordered upon the dangerous, before I finally came upon the truth. And the TRUTH is this! No matter what you may be suffering from, regardless of how feverish, weak or desperately ill you may feel,—NATURE WANTS TO SAVE YOU! Disease is merely Nature's effort to start performing the process of healing—the elimination of wastes and disease matters that clog up your tissue system. Listen to the instinctive advice of Nature unfailingly given to both man and animals! "Give me a chance to eliminate; to repair your bodily mechanism!" Take time to be "sick" for a few days or even weeks, and I will help you! "Remain still, quiet, rest, sleep and DON'T EAT!"

When you obstruct Nature's good intentions thru the use of man-made synthetic drugs—or continue eating more and more of the disease producing foods—or if the quantities of waste, mucus and poisons in your body are too much and too old—then Nature cannot help; and you must die just as animals do who fail to recuperate thru fasting alone. In fact it is thru this very method that Nature wipes out the weak, the degenerated ones who violated nature's laws of living, whether deliberately or innocently thru ignorance. The natural tendency of evolution seeks as a goal, not quantity but quality! It is truly indicative of how far man has degenerated thru wrong living, especially thru wrong eating.

The selection and preparation of his various foods, become immensely important factors of life when one recognizes that a large percentage of all mankind living today could not endure a long fast! You can learn more about these surprising facts in my book, the "MUCUSLESS DIET HEALING SYSTEM".° Without a corrective diet a perfect health CANNOT be attained thru modern miracle drugs or any form of accepted remedies or thru mechanical treatments. A supreme, absolute, Paradisical health—the way of infallible healing must be achieved thru, and is ruled by, the laws of diet. Man, like every living plant and organism matures and owes his existence to food. Man's health or his disease of every description, directly result from food intake. His state of mind may be a contributing factor, but the fall of mankind in the final analysis is "sin of diet". The real physiological cause of all evils, especially the physical ailments of mankind can be traced directly to the present day accepted diet of civilization. Having allowed your body to degenerate thru over-eating wrong, disease producing food, prayer alone will prove unavailing without a physical effort being made to correct your wrong living habits. Mankind's salvation and his return to the ideal prototype of the "perfect" normal being will require a complete healing from the "sins of the diet of civilization" as practiced today. Disease is internal uncleanliness acquired over all ages by wrong foods. My revelation of diseases and their healing thru corrective diet is based on proof and backed by experience and experiments conducted on my own body as well as thousands of patients at my Sanitarium in Switzerland during a period of over fifteen years. All methods of Natural treatments are indeed more or less cleansing, healing and even more or less rejuvenating, but fail to completely overcome the SOURCE—which is the direct cause of the "clogging-up" condition. A well selected "cleansing" diet consisting of fresh fruits and green leaf vegetables, makes it a distinct pleasure rather than a "painful" experience. The different kinds of food making many variations possible, the prescribed rest and relaxation are all indicated in each individual case and therefore must be especially selected to meet the varying situations. For example, a careful determination of the quantity of waste and poisons in the daily elimination of mucus now being dissolved and carried off by the blood stream should be recognized. The coated tongue and the sample specimen of urine, the putrid fecal matter are all tell-tale stories. The vital efficiency of the patient should not be obstructed, and therefore a "slowing-down" of the aggressive effect of elimination is advisable. The more time allowed for the body to throw off the stored up poisons, the less vitality will be required to do the work, and the more certain of success in the treatment! For example: where the case history shows that "drugs" have been used over a long period of time, it becomes extremely advisable to "slow-down" the aggressive effect of elimination thru the use of cooked foods—especially vegetables containing roughage,—such as found in beets, beet tops, spinach, celery, etc. If the "ailment" is at all remediable, Nature heals not only the disease, but the whole man! It may require as long as one to three years of systematically continued natural cleansing diets and fasting for the average "sick" person before the body is cleansed of "foreign matters". Assuring results will of course be noticed within the first few weeks. You may then see how the body is constantly eliminating waste from the urinary canal, the colon, the eyes, ears, nose and throat; from every pore of the skin over the entire surface of the body! You will observe how both "wet" and "dried" mucus, (dandruff, scaly formations in the nose, wax in the ear drums, for instance) is being continuously expelled. You will then readily agree with me when I state that all diseases of mankind, both mental and physical—ever since the beginning of our civilization has the same foundational cause—whatever the symptoms may be! It is without a single exception one and the same universal condition; a "one-ness" of all disease; and that is: Waste, foreign matter, excess mucus, and their related poisons, ie: stench (offensive odor) or "invisible waste". Everyone, no matter to what extent he may claim to enjoy "good health" has a latent sickness! A severe "shock" such as the so-called "cold" or "influenza" starts the elimination thruout the entire body. This attempted "house-cleaning" by Mother Nature should not be interfered with, either by continued eating or the use of drug suppressants. Nature should be permitted to eliminate this excess waste, often stored in the body since early childhood! Interference often results in producing "acute" and "chronic" diseases. It goes without saying that the process of elimination is not a pleasant experience, but how self-satisfying it is to know positively that you have averted a more severe stage of the illness that a postponement would have eventually made necessary. Man's mastery of disease will bring humanity closer to perfection of the human body. If you hope to achieve good health, freedom from pain and all illness, and the full enjoyment of a Paradisical existence, it can be obtained thru proper observance of Nature's laws, pertaining to the creation of man himself.

The truth of my statements are self-evident—and mankind will continue to go on and on, suffering never ending aches and pains, until the truth shall set him free. No one needs to live with disease —and freedom from disease has now become a reality. My "Mucusless Diet Healing System" has brought to all who would listen and heed, all of the information needed to banish illness and suffering from disease. Cleansing is basic for the correction and elimination of all disorders from which man suffers, caused thru the accumulation of poisons and congestion thru-out the entire body. Unusable and accumulated waste stored in the tissues cause degeneration and decay. When we stop feeding and cleanse our system, we allow the body to return to normalcy. "Magic cures", "witch-craft" or "miracle drugs" cannot possibly eliminate the cause of any disease. The "cleansing diet" is at the same time a "body building" diet—leaving the body free from the accumulation of toxic waste, brought about thru the eating of "mucus-forming" foods. Skin disorders and other conditions such as, boils. abscesses and carbuncles; Nature's untiring effort to eliminate excess waste and poisons will disappear quickly from the body. Correct foods, (fruits and green leaf vegetables) permit Nature to build a strong, healthy body; wrong foods produce a diseased body. We can eliminate all suffering, ailments and disease thru the physiological operations of diet. As the goal of the infallible true food of man you will find in Genesis 1-29 a biological law of eating. Foods, manufactured and prepared by man, only cause disease, troubles and sickness, and are therefore "wrong foods". Right foods, fresh fruits and green-leaf vegetables are healthy, divine foods, healing and diseaseless; paradisical living! Believing, knowing, having complete faith in these truthful facts and their scientific application, is the infallible principles of all healing, the REAL knowledge that must eventually result in the physiological salvation of mankind. Man today gets too much food —not too little! We must realize the limitations of the human digestive system.

I now have successfully solved the problem thru a scientifically correct system, and I can unequivocally state the following truth: "DISEASE is Nature's effort to rid the body of 'disease matters' and eliminate waste from the system".

The deeper causes of internal uncleanliness and its resulting constipation, can be definitely corrected and overcome thru my teachings, not merely relieved! This has proven to be the one sane, useable, and scientific Road to Regeneration. The simplicity and naturalness of these methods cannot help but appeal to the intelligent layman interested in self-betterment, both physical, mental and spiritual.

You now hold in your hands a scientific source of diet information; a cleansing diet nature intended for the use of man—a diet that can rid your system of disease-causing, poisonous filth—truly the discovery of the "Road to Health".

(FINIS)

—11—

PREFACE

I have been an Ehret devotee for the past twenty-five years and I shall remain so until the end of my days. My greatest desire is to share with others the wonderful results I have gained, both in physical and mental health.

The experiences outlined in the following article, MY ROAD TO HEALTH, are of course all true. Were I to continue re-writing these experiences for the next ten years, the wording and phrasing might be improved, but the truth must always remain the same. I shall always consider my experiences with the Ehret diet the greatest accomplishment of my entire life!

When I think of the benefits that could accrue to the human race were we to renounce the foods of present day civilization and return to a diet of natural, un-adulterated foods such as taught by Prof. Ehret, my heart becomes heavy and I find it almost more than I can bear. The problem, therefore, is, how to convince others of these truths. I can only hope that I have been the means of pointing the way even in some small degree.

It is the average person that I am anxious to reach so that they may be led, ever so gently, on to the right path in matters of diet. I consider the Mucusless Diet Healing System so great a benefaction to mankind, that I feel it should have all the publicity possible, not for monetary gain, but for more noble and humanitarian reasons, and the love of our fellow man.

Health is within everyone's grasp—all we need do is reach for it. Perhaps it will be difficult in the beginning; it might even take considerably longer than we would like, but in the end, our efforts will surely be crowned with the energy that radiates from a healthy body and which ultimately brings success and happiness.

Teresa Mitchell

MY ROAD TO HEALTH

by

TERESA MITCHELL

It all started many years ago in the war-torn country of Hungary. The many privations, frustrating experiences and abuses our family had been subjected to during the troubled times of the first World War had, undoubtedly, served to develop an intense desire on my part to overcome the conditions into which I, together with others of my class, had been tossed. When World War One finally ended, mother and myself were most fortunate in being presented with an opportunity to immigrate to this greatest of all countries, the United States of America. We gratefully embraced the chance and left for the land of our dreams just as fast as it was legally possible for us to do. America proved to be unbelievably wonderful—far beyond my most imaginative dreams.

Adjusting ourselves to American ways of living, but more especially adapting ourselves to American eating habits, was not particularly easy. The change from the meager rations of our war-time diet to the abundance of the American diet soon proved my physical undoing. During the war period our diet in Hungary was practically meatless and sugarless. Now in America I could have as much meat, pastries, sugar and dairy products that I wanted—just the kind of food I had been craving—without any restriction on quantities. This was America, the land of plenty—truly a land of milk and honey. I soon found my health declining. Continued illness led to consultations with doctors who informed me that, possibly the drastic change in food could be responsible. Fortunately for me, through the help of new found friends, I learned of the wonderful, free Public Libraries where many books on diet could be found. I avidly read most of them for they interested me greatly, particularly those dealing with vegetarian diets. Gradually, I began to apply many of the diet suggestions to my own eating habits. The results proved extremely gratifying, for unwittingly I had returned to my previous vegetarian diet. The first proof of good results was when I found that I no longed needed reading glasses, after having worn them for the previous three years. I joined a Hiking Club and learned to enjoy the great outdoors, climbing mountains and spending the day close to Nature's secrets. Our Hike Leader taught us common sense breathing exercises, during the frequent but short rest periods while we were on our hikes. At last I felt that I had discovered the right way for me to live. Surely, now, I would be most happy to live this way the remainder of my life. And then, most fortunately for me, I learned about a book called the *Mucusless Diet Healing System*, written by Prof. Arnold Ehret. I still treasure my copy of this marvelous book, whose dog-eared pages I still read and re-read (even after 27 years) and continue to find wonderful. This book was the real stepping stone to my Shangri-La of Health. This Shangri-La was not a place cloistered by tall mountains, reached only after grueling effort and hardship by only a few determined and courageous souls. No, on the contrary, my Shangri-La is readily accessible to everyone wanting to enter through its doors.

I soon learned that all I had heretofore read about health and diet was only partly right. But, now with my new knowledge, plus courage, faith and back-bone, perfect health was actually within my grasp and could be achieved through the understandable teachings contained in this remarkable book. Almost immediately I felt the author's sincerity and accepted every word of his teachings. Instinctively I knew that this time I was on the right track. After many months of following the "Transition Diet" as taught by Ehret, the cleansing I achieved startled me. Yes, the effectiveness of the diet was unquestionable. A miracle in healing had taken place right under my very eyes. For instance, a goiter which had already become annoyingly obvious on my neck, completely disappeared! I could not believe it possible to feel any better than I now felt. Various minor symptoms, almost too numerous to mention, likewise disappeared.

Two years had passed since I first began the transition diet and

—14—

by now I truly relished all of the foods that were allowed me. I earnestly followed the exercises given in the book as well as developing some of my own. A fine breathing exercise, which I discovered, helped me overcome the weakness that often accompanies a drastic diet change. The time was now approaching when the final great step for complete healing, as taught by Prof. Ehret, should be taken. The decision was not easy. I began questioning myself, "Do I dare take it?" "Why go further since I really feel fine now." "I must be physically all right for it has been a long time since I have had even a 'simple' cold". As I kept arguing with myself, strange thoughts, as well as doubts, came into my mind. "Suppose the author was wrong—it is barely possible that he might be mistaken in his conclusions." While Ehret taught 'man's food is fruits and green leaf vegetables' how could anyone possibly exist on such a monotonous diet? "Is my will-power strong enough?"

I began to discuss Prof. Ehret's teachings with others who, like myself, were interested in regaining health through diet. Some had made an attempt but not one among them went all the way through with the diet. "It takes too much will-power," I was told by some, while others said, "You'll dry up," or "Your bones will become brittle through lack of calcium." "Modern civilization makes it impossible." Others, apparently more kindly, admonished, "Why do it— is it not enough that you are healthy now?" "You will be all alone in your belief—no one will understand you." How I longed to take my problems directly to Prof. Ehret, but at the very pinnacle of success he had, unfortunately, met with a fatal accident. After a long and careful review of the 'pros and cons' I came to the decision that my life was my own and I would do with it as I saw fit. I seemed to realize that until I had thoroughly tried Ehret's teachings I could know no real feeling of success. All fear left as soon as my decision was made and I decided to confide in no one. My goal was to "taste of Paradise" as Ehret had promised. This experimenting with restricted diets had now been going on for a period of years, and ironically enough, during the entire period, the only jobs available to me were in restaurants— either Cashier, Food Checker or Waitress.

My decision made, I started out early one morning with determination in my heart. I halfway expected everything and everyone to be different—but upon my arrival at work everyone and everything was the same as always—the tantalizing smells of frying bacon and "ham and eggs," the urn full of steaming coffee and the trays heavily laden with food. The few early morning, sleepy-eyed women, the men patrons in grimy coats and their work-stained overalls—all were the same as before. As a matter of fact, only one thing was actually different—and that was my mental attitude which no one seemed to notice—not immediately, nor for a while at least, that is to say.

A DIFFICULT FIRST WEEK

It was no easy matter to live up to this decision of remaining on a strict fruit diet until complete healing of my body was accomplished. Over and over again, I had to remind myself of the blessings I had hoped to gain and only by holding a mental picture of success in front of me, more times than I care to admit, the first week finally passed. I daresay, this first week was the hardest part of the entire venture. Having no precedent to go by as to the right amount of fruit that I should eat at one meal, I did a little experimenting. Fortunately, watermelons were in season and I soon found them to be more filling than most other fruits. Co-workers and friends began to notice the monotony of my meals, and I found it difficult to keep my secret. Finally, I decided to confide in the manager and he understandably told others about it. From then on I was a "freak" among the employees but, fortunately, it did not bother me too much.

My previous years on vegetarian diets proved advantageous, having conditioned me, more or less, for an exclusive fruitarian diet, yet, it is true, I lost considerable weight. The vegetarian diet had accomplished a lot of good results in the elimination of toxic encumbrances and waste matter and the toxin-producing meat and dairy products had no part in my diet for the past number of years. However, frequent expectoration continued for a long time while on the fruit regime, and I also noticed considerable elimination of

—16—

stringy mucus accompanying my stool. Yet there were many indications of general improvement in my health which gave me increased determination to go on with my experiment.

The skin on my face which had seemed to sag after the first ten days or two weeks became firm and smooth again after a period of a month's time. My eyes became clear and bright and a new feeling of exhilaration came over me. This was something I had seldom experienced, if at all. I decided I must be making progress.

The grape season was now on hand and I found all varieties of grapes to be a satisfying food. While Muscat grapes seemed to be the most pleasing and satisfying to me, I enjoyed any kind of grapes. I soon discovered that it required only about an hour for fruits to digest and I therefore, ate whenever I would feel the gnawing pangs of hunger. But, and this is extremely important, I learned that even fruits have a harmful reaction if one overeats of them! Nature has a very subtle way of letting us know when we have eaten enough.

A WORKABLE DIET

This new habit of eating whenever I felt hunger pangs proved difficult to manage during working hours. When I thought that no one was looking I would sneak a bite from an apple or other fruit which I had hidden near the cash register. The manager soon put an end to this surreptitious eating but he kindly suggested that I help myself to whatever fruit might be in the refrigerator. Needless to say, this made life much easier. What was most amazing to me was that I had not become weakened through this strict fruit diet. While I had been forewarned that I might even become bed-fast for a time, the "weakness" I had been led to expect failed to materialize. I did not miss one single day from my work.

I love to sing and on frequent occasions I have been told that I have a fairly good voice so during the previous two years I had been taking vocal lessons. After three months on this rigid diet my teacher remarked about a decided change that was taking place in in the quality of my voice as well as decided changes in my general appearance and personality. It seemed that I had more breath and better control, and that my voice had more resonance—in fact, had become much clearer. I was thrilled with this progress but still hesitated about revealing my diet to my teacher for I enjoyed the moral strength that keeping this secret seemed to give me.

Even after six months of my exclusive fruit diet I still had not reached the point where, according to Prof. Ehret's teachings, all obstacles would be swept aside. Living in a rooming house, completely alone, with Mother, my only living relative in this country, thousands of miles away (she had remained in Ohio when I came to California), I was finding it a difficult fight. Mother and I corresponded regularly, yet, I never revealed my diet to her for fear of being discouraged by her. Encouragement was what I most needed at this point of the experiment. Loneliness was probably the most difficult of all the obstacles I had to battle. I tried to keep my mind occupied through reading and planning the things I would like to do after reaching my goal with the diet. Despite the many friends I made with almost everyone with whom I came in contact, that strange loneliness still persisted. With the arrival of Fall came apple time. I fondly recall the delicious Jonathan apples which helped to vary my diet. A large sized Jonathan made a complete meal in itself.

By this time I had been living on the fruitarian diet for about nine months and many encouraging and wonderful things had taken place. For at least the past two months I had felt like a new born babe. How I wanted to shout this message from the house tops. "This must be the way God intended man to live. Why won't people accept these teachings—or at least try for themselves, so that they might enjoy the truth." In my enthusiasm I dreamed of having a whole colony of people living this Paradisiacal life. To my young mind this was the answer to all of the ills of humanity and loneliness as well.

My skin texture became like that of a baby. The natural red of my lips no longer made the use of lipstick necessary. My eyes were clear and bright at all times. In fact, my entire being was gradually

—18—

taking on a complete change. Yes, even my disposition changed for the better and a natural display of quick temper had given way to a quiet philosophic attitude toward all people and their daily problems. Fears, with which I was formerly plagued, were gradually disappearing. My thinking had changed completely. People constantly remarking about the natural and spontaneous smile that lighted my face. There was no effort needed to produce it. This wonderful feeling of exhilaration became part of my life. It was my first conscious thought upon awakening every morning.

THE FIRST CLEANSING

Then the first great event happened. One night, after a supper of grapes, I was awakened by a sensation of fullness in my throat. I had no particular feeling of nausea or pain, but upon reaching the bathroom I threw up large quantities of a sticky, clear substance. After this ordeal was over I felt a new sense of well-being come over me. New strength and power seemed to fill my whole being. I thought, this must be the great final cleansing that Prof. Ehret taught us to expect. However, it was only a forerunner of two more similar experiences before the long expected day arrived.

During this period of cleansing and elimination many interesting things took place—in fact, too many to enumerate here. One of the most outstanding facts, I think, was the complete absence of fatigue. My work required that I remain constantly on my feet for eight hours, and yet after a full day's work I felt just as fresh as though I had not worked at all. The only way I knew that rest was required by my body was a feeling of drowsiness. Upon arriving home I usually took a short nap, after which I was ready for my vocal studies at the studio. My rest at night was complete and undisturbed, for I seldom dreamed. Upon awakening there was that indescribable clear-headedness which must be experienced in order to be understood and appreciated. No stimulants, such as coffee or tea, were needed to get me in good humor for the days work. Thinking was becoming increasingly easier and I was actually becoming witty. In fact, I had never been aware of this gift in my adopted

English language. I felt proud of my ability to give back a quick answer, as well as a ready come-back to "small" talk. My powers of concentration had become more acute. In fact, neither noises or confusion could distract my thinking. My shyness and reticence were being replaced by poise.

Many daily temptations had to be overcome, such as when an urgent desire for foods that I knew to be harmful, presented itself, I learned through repetition that the sooner I told myself NO the easier it became to say NO the next time. A realization soon came to me that keeping my mind occupied with other things, instead of permitting thoughts of food to form, helped increase my will-power.

My residence was close to the restaurant so that I could walk to and from work. There was one exceptionally steep hill to climb which would invariably cause me to puff and pant. One afternoon on my way home I felt inspired to create a poem. As the sentences took form I became deeply engrossed in thought when suddenly I noticed I had climbed more than half way up the hill, yet I had felt no exertion whatever. It was as though I had been walking on level ground and I could scarcely believe what was happening. I concluded that I must have been so engrossed in the poem that I forgot about my body. This, then, was an opportune time to make a test, so I decided to return to the bottom of the hill and walk up again, this time giving no thought to the poem. What I discovered was unbelievable. I felt as though my body had no weight at all. Here was I, ascending this steep incline, which in all probability is at least sixty percent grade, without the slightest feeling of fatigue whatsoever. I am sure that I could have easily run all the way up, and I would have tried it too, except I feared I would cause consternation among the puffing and panting pedestrians. It was difficult for me to restrain myself from stopping my fellow pedestrians and telling them all about it. "I must be at the very gates of Shangri La," I thought to myself, "To think that diet could do all this."

After my enthusiasm calmed down a bit and after considerable thought, I decided to tell certain people whom I believed might understand. While some marvelled at my will-power, others simply refused to believe my story and still others felt that while it might be a good thing for me, it surely would not be the right procedure for them to follow. It was discouraging to have people say, "You are young—it is your youth." "Yes", I answered, "I am young. Just how young do you think I am?" "Well, you can't be more than sixteen." When I gave my age as twenty-six they were incredulous.

Within myself I knew all was well and I continued eating my fruit meals. Other seemingly unexplainable experiences followed. My feeling of well-being was boundless—I knew I was now completely restored to perfect health—I had arrived at my long hoped-for goal. No aches and pains, no physical discomfort of any kind, no headaches, no colds. This might be a good time to mention another of the "experiences" that were occurring to me. My menstrual periods only occurred at six months intervals, and when they did come, I felt no nervous reaction or mental depression and absolutely no pain whatsoever. Their duration was very short.

Words seem inadequate to describe the perfect state of well-being I was now privileged to experience. Sound in body, health and mind, I considered myself fortunate indeed. The thrill of being alive was so intense that I felt this great thrill must be shared with others, for to keep it a secret was surely a sin. No doubt about it, I was an entirely different person, living in a private Paradise all my own, wonderful beyond description—calm, serene and the few talents with which God had endowed me, greatly improved.

It was my looks, my general appearance, which most certainly showed the greatest improvement. Despite a loss of twenty-five pounds, I, by no means, looked "skinny." I was slender in body, yes, but my face was gently rounded and my skin was like that of a baby. I was bubbling over with happiness at all times and a glow of radiance seemed to emanate from me, since people continually remarked about it. Complete calmness and a feeling of confidence, like the confidence a small child must feel sitting in the lap of his mother, safe from outside harm, invaded me. Perhaps I had better describe it as sitting in the lap of God, with a small inner voice

—21—

reassuring me that I was at last free from all disease. So long as my blood stream remained clean and pure, and my tissues were no longer clogged with the encumbrances of foreign waste matter, no outside germs could attack and harm my physical body. This was a staggering realization, to say the least, and I wanted to make the most of it.

In discussing my experiences with others I was not too surprised to learn that they had tried to live on the Ehret diet but failed. Either through lack of faith or lack of will-power, possibly both, they quit too soon. They had missed the great realization, so important to one's future life. Those who failed probably brand the Ehret teachings as unsound, but, so far as I am concerned, everything taught by the author in his "Mucusless Diet Healing System" is true. I have personally proven that every statement contained in Prof. Ehret's book is based on a solid foundation of undeniable truth. This, then is the kind of health the average person cannot even conceive of, with every organ and cell of the body completely free and able to function as God intended it should, without obstructions of any kind. Probably Prof. Ehret was the only man in recent history to achieve this perfect health.

I have proven to my complete satisfaction the human body does not need the scientifically prepared foods and complicated diets that present day civilization has come to accept as absolutely essential for health. I now know that the human body, after it has been cleansed of all the dross refuse (waste encumbrances that our modern diet leaves in every cell and in every drop of the blood stream) can exist on fruits alone and be marvelously healthy. And I have found that even the youngest infant must first go through a diet of cleansing before he can be fed on this "diet of Paradise," as the author called it.

Prof. Ehret's mucusless diet truly possesses the potentialities of saving this mixed-up world of ours with a rebirth of spirituality difficult to conceive even in the twentieth century. All of the five senses became keener:—clearer vision, brighter colors, sounds, even whispers became distinctly audible, and re-awakened taste buds made flavors tastier and scents more keen. Small wonder I still inwardly weep when I think of the misery, pain, fear, plus all of the other trials and tribulations which make living so difficult. I became heart sick when I watched people carrying trays laden with at least five times as much food as the capacity of their stomach. Their poor, overworked organs lacked sufficient vitality to dispose of this excess quantity of waste. Small wonder they were continually "sick"—small wonder they were always tired and worn out.

Today, after a span of twenty-seven years, my faith in the efficacy of Ehret's "Mucusless Diet Healing System" is stronger than it ever was during my younger days of experimenting. At the age of fifty-three, I am proudly beginning to admit my age. For years I had fibbed about it, especially to my employers. Now, my neighbors and co-workers look at me with great surprise. I am told that I should never admit to being more than thirty-six or seven, at the most. My skin (I must admit, at the risk of seeming to brag) still has the unwrinkled smoothness of a much younger woman. My hair is in excellent condition. I have retained a youthful streamlined figure. My voice, which I use a great deal as a soloist, is still young and vibrant. I keep up an extensive vocal repertoire. I still enjoy the zest, capacity and strength for work. I do all my own housework and carry on a seven or eight hour job, outside my home. I take care of such duties as two growing sons and a husband. In my spare time I try my hand at writing. I am completely without aches or pains of any kind, although I have been going through the difficult period of menopause. However, the generally accepted symptoms that plague the average woman during this period of life, have had very slight effects on me. I have not had "shots," pills or tonics—in fact, I have had no need to even seek the advice of a physician. My medicine cabinet is still free of pills, physics or tonics, nor do I use creams and beauty preparations.

Needless to say, I do not wander off the straight and narrow path as laid down by Prof. Ehret in his wonderful book which, I am sure, does not need my testimonial for it has stood on its own merits for many years. Over a hundred thousand persons have already read the book and many must believe its teachings just as I do. But,

—23—

may I emphasize just one point, and it is this: Whoever desires to become a disciple of Ehret's teachings should himself attain a complete healing. Then, and then only, is he competent to teach the principles of "How to Control One's Health" through Fasting and Diet, without fear of unknown disease that might be lurking in the tissues and blood-stream of the body.

Only this can give man's soul and mind the freedom Nature intended us to possess.

PART II

BUILD YOUR OWN ROAD TO HEALTH

Everyone can create his own perfect health regardless of age or condition. This might seem like a bold statement to make, but, I assure you, it is true. If you are willing to make the effort, to learn to have faith and to teach yourself perseverance, *you can have perfect health.*

Rejuvenation is within your reach: a life full of action, accomplishment and, most certainly, full of the joy of living; a sane and well balanced life that affords no time for frustrations nor neuroses.

All through the history of mankind, old age has been pictured as the burdensome years, the years of decline, of senility—and ailments. But this no longer has to be so. Actually, the most rewarding and productive period of your life should be during these advanced years. This time of maturity should be spent doing the type of work requiring the experience that only a mature mind possesses. By this time, too, a certain amount of economic stability has been established. But, alas, in our present so-called civilized condition, with but few exceptions, we are too senile and too ill to enjoy fully this wonderful freedom and security. Too many of us are relegated to park benches, hoping to relieve our aching bones and throbbing joints by basking in the sunshine.

The crippling diseases of old age need never occur nor should degenerative diseases be taken for granted at any age. But, unfortunately, Man continually tries unnatural methods to heal himself and in that lies his downfall.

Fortunately, Arnold Ehret, in his °"Mucusless Diet Healing System," teaches methods in complete harmony with natural laws—methods which he followed to heal himself completely. He points out that Nature's laws are immutable. Man must first learn to subjugate himself and then fully cooperate with them if he would enjoy physical and mental harmony.

Anyone seriously contemplating the truly inspiring journey to perfect health through the pages of Ehret's "Mucusless Diet Healing System" must realize that it requires careful study and intelligent judgment. The lessons contained in the book must be studied thoroughly and many times over so that the thoughts of this great health teacher become familiar. There are several very important points you must remember.

If you are suffering from an ailment pronounced "incurable," you cannot possibly expect the same immediate results as someone suffering from a minor ailment. Age, too, is necessarily an important factor. The same reaction cannot be expected by a person in his seventies as an individual in the thirties, twenties or younger.

You must condition yourself in both body and mind to achieve the best results. For example, the three-time-a-day meat-eater should not suddenly deprive himself of all meat products. This would prove a tremendous shock physically as well as mentally. It would be much wiser for you to cut down on food portions over a period of months and then gradually eliminate one meat meal (preferably breakfast). After a few months you can eliminate the lunch meat dish and then you can leave off meat at dinner. Substitute a cooked vegetable plate which you really enjoy in place of the meat dish. This tapering off system can be just as successfully applied in eliminating coffee, tea, carbohydrates, eggs, dairy products, etc.

A tapering off system serves many purposes. First of all, it begins the disciplining of the mind which is so essential to success in this undertaking. Secondly, it begins the gradual elimination of the acids and pus in the system. Thirdly, it reduces the size of the stomach, if the suggestion not to overeat is followed.

FROM WRONG TO RIGHT

The transition diet, set forth in the book, is just what its name implies: a transition from a previous wrong way of eating to the correct, new way. The most important thing accomplished through this new regimen is the elimination of accumulated wastes with its resultant healing. First the tottering structure is slowly and gradually torn down and the debris removed to make room for the new and modern structure.

Many students believe it is ncessary to eat larger portions of fruits and vegetables when on the transition diet since it does not have the heavier consistency of today's conventional diet. But, this is not so. You actually need less fruits and vegetables since they contain more food value. You will be surprised at the small amount of food your body really needs to nourish itself. If you eat more food than you need, this surplus food must be eliminated and so your organs of elimination may be over-worked. Gas may form if too much fruit is eaten at one time, and fruit mixed with starches tends to form gas.

It would be wise for you to eat slowly and *you should never eat unless hungry.* Nature has a very definite signal by which she lets us know when the meal is over. You must learn to heed this signal. Often acid pangs are mistakenly thought to be hunger pangs. (There is a similarity.) These false hunger pangs will disappear as the surplus acids are eliminated. Acid pangs come and go while hunger pangs persist.

Some people complain about leaving the table unsatisfied after an all-fruit meal. This is understandable for back of all of us is a lifetime of wrong habits that require time to change. You must actually make a conscious effort to change your ideas on food and nutrition. One habit that must be broken is the one of expecting a "stuffy" or "full" feeling at the end of a meal. Relish the new kind of food in your thoughts and I am sure you will soon like it well enough to look forward to your next meal.

You must not become discouraged. Check for improvements daily to encourage yourself. In a younger person, within a week's time after starting on the transition diet, a definite improvement will be noted: the skin is clearer, the eyes are brighter, a general feeling of lightness develops and the desire for more activity increases. There is a definite psychological lift in all this. One is constantly looking forward to improvements in one's health. The all-absorbing fear of being struck down by numberless degenerative diseases is gradually erased from the mind.

CONTROLLING WEIGHT LOSS

Don't be alarmed because you lose weight. "Weight is disease" and all of the old diseased substances must go. However, you should not lose weight too rapidly. If you do, add a baked potato or some melba toast to your meals for a while. Cottage cheese will also help check too rapid a weight loss.

You should continue with the transition diet until a feeling of well-being is established. This can only take place after the greater part of the waste encumbrances are eliminated. The length of time required to attain complete healing will depend on your age and physical condition. When you consider that your present state is the result of a whole life time of wrong eating, you should not begrudge a few years spent in healing yourself.

Most women are ingenious with foods and the menus in the transition diet will not present a problem for they can be changed to suit one's own tastes. The most important thing to remember when preparing a menu is simplicity. Seasoning foods is not necessary. Learn to bring out the natural flavors of foods by baking or braising in a small amount of water and either pure olive oil or another good vegetable oil. We are extremely fortunate in being supplied with delicious fresh frozen foods all year around. Salad lettuce is available even during the winter months in most parts of the country and fresh cabbage, carrots and celery make a delicious combination. Many salad variations can be built on just these few vegetables. Try shredding carrots and adding freshly cooked or canned young peas, making a dressing with the cooked vegetable juice or a mixture of honey and lemon juice. Experience will show you many other similar combinations.

You should not try the complete fruit fast until you are quite certain that all of the dangerous waste matter has been eliminated from your body. Fruit is a relentless eliminator of diseased substances. Many of us could not possibly undergo this severe type of housecleaning because of our physical condition. Vegetables, both naturally raw and cooked, work thoroughly but much more slowly and gently. The fruit diet in itself is the "proof of the pudding." If you are able to live on it comfortably, without any untoward reactions, you are healed. This reminds me of the case of a middle aged person who really tried to prepare himself over a period of three or four years for an exclusive fruit diet. Unfortunately, the "cleansing" was not complete for the sinuses still contained mucus which had not been completely emptied for years. Apparently there was also some pus in his system clamoring for release. His experience was very unpleasant for he became poisoned by his own dross. He could have avoided this had he made certain that his system was free of the old and poisonous substances. You can make certain by observing the reaction to a fruit fast of no more than twenty-four hours duration. If the result is a severe headache, dizziness, bad breath, thickly coated tongue, increased mucus discharge from throat and nose, it is quite certain that you are not ready for a pure fruit diet.

Our tongue is the "magic mirror" in which, as Ehret teaches, we can watch for symptoms during the fast. It is a definite indication of the true condition of the tissues as well as the internal organs of the abdominal cavity. When the internal organs are completely healthy, the tongue takes on a permanent healthy pink color. Observe the tongues of animals; they are always the same healthy pink. The breath should be absolutely pure and inoffensive. There should be no acid or pus condition. All this is plainly revealed in the "magic mirror."

During the process of elimination, the skin becomes loose and even wrinkled but this is a natural result in everyone, regardless of age, during the healing crises. The natural foods now being consumed, perhaps for the first time during the person's life, start working to improve and rebuild. Nature wisely takes advantage of this situation and begins "house-cleaning." Then after the sticky mucus is thoroughly eliminated and a clean, rebuilt blood stream is present, the tissues will regain their elasticity. New and healthy cells of the tissues will fill with oxygen and puff themselves up proudly like tiny feather pillows. The daily improvement will be so obvious that you will surely be thrilled to see it. The texture of your skin will completely change and your body will take on a youthfulness that will surprise you. Your muscles will become firm and resilient and the joy of being alive will fill you with a desire to give your message to the whole world.

PATIENCE AND PERSISTENCE

It is much better to take your time about this business of healing. It is the most important step you can take in this life. The results are surely worth while and all you need do is use some common sense *and follow Nature's rules.* If you start on the road to health the Ehret way, persist until the complete healing. It will provide the essential moral support as nothing else possibly can. Whatever you do, DON'T give up too soon for you may well be almost within sight of success. As we travel the road of Ehretism, we are not only helping ourselves, but we are also instrumental, through our example, in establishing a new way of life for hundreds of others.

— FINIS —

INTERNAL CLEANLINESS

as based on the teachings of Arnold Ehret

by

FRED S. HIRSCH

HEALTH is the inevitable result of strict obedience to God's physical and natural laws—HEALTH is happiness in the body! Almost automatically, one turns to the holy scriptures for time honored, proven quotations for reaffirmation and confirmation of this contention. In I Cor. 139:17 we read: "If a man defy the temple of God, him shall God destroy". Are we to doubt that God intended for man's body to be the "temple"? "If ye know these things, happy are ye if ye do them". John 13:17. And again, in I Cor. 6:20 "Glorify God in your body and spirit, which are God's". Can any one deny the meaning as expressed so clearly and unmistakenly in 2 Cor. 7-1: "Let us cleanse ourselves from all filthiness of the flesh and spirit" The word "spirit" is derived from the Greek word, "spiro" meaning breath or air we breathe. Evidently there were victims of "bad breath" in Biblical times, since they were exhorted to "cleanse the spirit". If the human body is kept in comfortable environments under natural dietetic laws and furnished solely with foods God planned for human nourishment—there is little doubt that man could continue to live indefinitely, free from disease, aches and pains. But man-made food substitutes and all foods grown in chemically treated soils, cause nutritional deficiency; result—the human organisms take on illness and disease. The application of inorganic fertilizers forces the soil to produce larger crops, thereby increasing the farmer's income; but only at the expense of the ultimate consumer who must eventually suffer the consequences thru the eating of these worthless, health-destroying foods. How we manage to exist at all; living in over-crowded cities with fellow men,—themselves the product of this faulty generation,—breathing foul, putrid air poisoned by gases belching forth from factory chimneys which joins the exhaust from millions of gasoline powered autos and motor trucks; "over-eating", mostly chemicalized food

—31—

substitutes from which all natural minerals and vitamins have been completely robbed and replaced with laboratory concoctions; drinking heavily chlorinated water which right now is being threatened by the authorities with compulsory fluorine treatment, and who knows how many more man-made chemicals? This continued air and water pollution will eventually succeed in canceling any progress science hopefully may achieve towards deferring old age. Tobacco smoke, air pollution and chemical poisons daily enter our body and directly cause premature old age.

Man's first food must have been fruits and uncooked green-leaf vegetables (fire had not as yet been invented—remember?)—his beverage was sparkling-fresh, pure uncontaminated water, from rippling brook or running stream. So it is plain to see that man by nature is a fruit-eating animal, and therefore fairly safe to claim that fruit and green leaf vegetables should constitute the main portion of our food intake. Were man willing to strictly follow and obey this fundamental and natural dietetic law, it would cause no surprise to find centenarians able to care for themselves without Medicare!—the rule rather than the exception. Unfortunately, continued violation of Nature's inviolable dietary laws carries with it certain and definite suffering. Clogging up of the "human machine", thru undigested, surplus quantities of food—cause a continual and gradual decline in our activity and the slowing down of vitality. The plea of ignorance is unacceptable and every violator of Nature's basic dietary laws must pay the penalty.

Present day custom of eating fruits as a dessert, or as a supplementary part of the meal carries with it a definite dietetic hazard. The digestion of ripened fruits starts immediately and is absorbed by the blood stream, with practically no drain on the vital forces. Contrariwise, meat and potatoes representing today's "mixtures" require hours for digestion. When fresh fruit juices enter the scene, gases rapidly form, bloating occurs and often a light form of "food poisoning" results. Fruits and undigested foods do not blend harmoniously and it would be wise to wait at least twenty minutes or longer after eating before following with fresh fruits. Because of this knowledge we can be forewarned and proceed properly. Fruits, especially tree ripened fruits eaten directly from the tree or vine (if at all possible), represent the "invisible knife" of Nature's surgery; loosening the mass of internal waste and poisons, often hardened and clinging to the walls of intestines for years—the direct source and cause of disease. We now know the secret of internal cleansing! Thru this very ability to thoroughly "cleanse"; a diet of fresh fruit could be harmful for the seriously ill individual. The too rapid elimination of quantities of poisonous waste materials, when thrown into the bloodstream carrying out nature's method of "cleansing" places too heavy a burden on the patient's vitality and the already overtaxed depurating organs; resulting in possible systemic disturbances. Because of lowered vitality, the body finds it now impossible to cope with the additional burden. Used with understanding and common sense, fruit can be considered as entirely safe, in fact, together with fasting it provides the only true method of a complete return to normal health. With the use of cooked and baked vegetables, leaving off fruit entirely from the diet until such time as the patient's vitality has increased, the heavily encumbered sick individuals will thus undergo a less strenuous "cleansing"—and then gradually make the change-over to a fruit diet in accordance with the patient's physical condition. This explains why we stress again and again that caution must prevail. Complete knowledge is necessary and a more comprehensive and detailed explanation of these all important principals are contained in Arnold Ehret's Mucusless Diet Healing System.° Fruits are man's natural food and their ability to cleanse the blood and tissues of foreign matters cannot be equalled. The average home is equipped with modern food blenders and juice extractors which make it possible to enjoy the benefits of fresh juices. All juices, both fresh fruit and vegetable juice are recognized dissolvers of disease producing hardened-fecal matter clinging to the entire intestinal tract; waste encumbrances which often remain in pockets of the intestines for years, and in fact are never completely evacuated even by the individual who boasts of "a daily bowel-movement". The juice of fresh crushed grapes, oranges, grapefruit, pineapple, prune, apricot and apple juice are almost in-dispensable during the healing process, for they must be recognized as Nature's own internal cleansers, as well as a source of life giving energy. Disease in every form is an accumulation of unelimated waste and foreign matter which must first be eliminated before the sick can return to normal health, free from illness of every kind! Disease itself consists of both a local and general congestion of any part or organ of the body which is unable to function normally be-cause of encumbrances and accumulated wastes. The name given the illness derives from the location in the system or the organ affected—the direct cause is the same!

Often the entire colon becomes overloaded — the descending colon actually impacted with decaying, putrid, waste matter finds itself unable to function, and a gradual backing-up of poisons in-to the vital depurating organs of the body (ie: liver, kidneys, stomach, lungs) interferes with their normal functioning. Disease cannot truthfully be said to result from external conditions, disease is created within the body—wrong foods and improper food com-binations,—excessive food intake,—a seemingly total disregard of Nature's laws—or at best total ignorance! Health must depend on a perfectly natural balance being kept thru proper assimilation and elimination; internal cleanliness! Even the very purest of food can disturb this balance if more is eaten than the body can assimilate, and the answer to discomfort from "over-eating" is—"Fast" All that is necessary is to pass up the next meal or two, give the body a chance to regain its natural balance!

This accumulated mass of age-old, stored-up waste, lodged in the tissues, is what Arnold Ehret called, "your latent disease" Eventually it becomes the source of "active" disease, and accumu-lated wastes are eliminated thru such minor ailments as the "com-mon cold"—influenza (the flu)—dysentery or a fever. It is then that the habit of "over-eating" if not discontinued, will cause the over-worked devitalized organs to "break-down" and normal functioning slows-down or ceases altogether. Vital, eliminative and depurating organs,—bowels, kidney, lungs and skin are constantly under pres-sure. Not only are they abused — but other vital parts of our

-34-

body, ie: stomach, liver, heart, eyes, ears and sinuses are also over-worked. Crankiness, mental depression, irritation, bad breath, ca-tarrhal conditions and a lack of energy can be more or less directly traced to excessive eating and particularly, wrong food combina-tions.

The undernourished persons are not necessarily found among the very poor. An extremely simple, low-cost diet provides sufficient life-giving nourishment; but the well-to-do individuals more often are victims of malnutrition! The "anti-poverty program" is not the final answer to this problem! Malnutrition can more often result from ex-cessive eating rather than from a "starvation diet!" The over-worked body lacks the vitality necessary to handle the tremendous load im-posed upon it thru over-eating! Conformity to accepted social cus-toms; lack of individual will-power, or just plain ignorance results in man willfully clogging his wonderful self-sustaining, self-healing hu-man machine with an unbelievable amount of excess food and drink! This continual failure to heed nature's repeated warning,—and merely paying lip-service to these doctrines thru self-sympathy, worry, depression, resentment—bring on eventual chronic invalid-ism. Man is slow to learn the lessons of experience; the absolute necessity of internal cleanliness! One would think that most people know how to maintain good health! After failing to heed Nature's warning he wonders why his sick condition exists! For complete restoration and maintenance of perfect health,—the foods needed are fresh fruits and green-leaf vegetables, a fact which Arnold Ehret continually stresses in his book; foods that do *not* deposit waste encumbrances; but actually cleanse the system of poisonous wastes thru natural elimination! Make a practice of eating the foods that *like* you—not those *you* like to eat! Only thru a thorough inter-nal cleansing from waste and related poisons can the desired goal of natural, normal health be obtained. Internal cleansing, thru a fruit diet and fasting are natural methods of procedure according to Ehret's philosophy.

When over-eating has finally brought about pain and illness, what could be more sensible than ridding the body of these waste encumbrances? Certainly neither ignoring or deploring the illness can effectively remove the cause. Every effort must be concentrated on removing and correcting the real trouble. "Cleanliness" it is said is "next to Godliness" which clearly and unmistakably means, cleanliness—internally, externally and eternally! Man can never return to normal health, nor can he remain well with his bodily system over-loaded and clogged-up thru retained poisonous waste!

The "mucus-forming" foods are known to be meat, eggs, dairy products, all starchy foods; (dried beans, mashed potatoes, gravies and refined cereals, to name but a few)—while the natural "cleansing" life-giving foods are fresh fruits and green-leaf vegetables. Starchy vegetables when used during the transition period should be thoroughly baked until all starch content is completely dextrinized. Vegetable salads both natural and cooked play an important part in the internal cleansing process. Salads containing "roughage" i.e.: celery, grated carrots, cole slaw, spinach, beets; are the "intestinal broom" so-named by Ehret for cleansing ability. And don't forget— the whole body must be cleansed,—not merely the diseased parts, and this cleansing must take place where the disease actually exists, i.e.: on the inside of the body! Hot and cold applications, body massage and heat-lamps are accepted modalities for relieving pain and building up muscular strength, and should be used for this purpose when necessary. With every organ functioning normally, the human body becomes a thing of beauty, joy and happiness; takes on strength, energy and mental alertness—becomes a wholesome clean, strong, healthy system, able to express physically and spiritually man's mission on earth!

CURATIVE FOODS

We hope that we have firmly established by now that natural foods, ie: fruit and green-leaf vegetables contain all of the necessary life building elements as well as cleansing qualities. If you are striving to maintain or regain normal health, limit your meals as much as possible to these foods. Should a marked disturbance take place during the period of "cleansing" merely stop eating fresh fruits and un-cooked vegetables and for a few days eat only cooked, baked vegetables. To enjoy life to its fullest extent, all rich, heavy, undigestible, highly seasoned foods that have clogged the system with wastes and encumbrances during the entire life period, must be discontinued. Have FAITH in the tremendous healing power of Nature, for faith is a most important factor in the healing program. Know exactly what you have set out to accomplish and let nothing interfere with your determination to succeed. The complete and thorough cleansing of the intestinal tract brings an unexpected, inflow of physical and mental strength. This astonishing truth that strength actually results from internal cleanliness rather than from food now hopefully dawns upon the sufferer who slowly begins to admit that eating excessive quantities of food—clog, weaken and disease the body —dull and depress the mind! The age-old belief that "the more rich food we eat the more strength we receive" becomes a fallacy! Ehret considered fasting almost indispensable for the final overcoming of all chronic conditions. Enemas are often indicated and in certain cases prove effective. For example: during a fast, and even during the "transition period", the bowel evacuation contains sticky, stringy mucus difficult for normal elimination and it is here that enemas prove helpful. Physical exercises combining stretching, and tensing movements, simple movements of the arms and legs are a daily must!

Primitive man would forego eating whenever ill at ease, but his modern counterpart evidently prefers to sacrifice almost anything else! Primitive man instinctively knew enough to remove causes—modern man ignores and even takes drugs to suppress causes. Sick or injured animals instinctively fast, refusing to eat until completely recovered. Search as you will,—modern civilization offers no better remedy than Nature's time proven method—the fast —and the observance of nature's dietetic laws; fruits and vegetables. We lose our appetite during illness yet modern practice is to "feed for strength", depleting precious vital energy urgently needed to throw off the illness! It was Hippocrates, the father of medicine who stated 2000 years ago; "the more you feed a sick man, the more you harm him". Unfortunately, only a few of his modern disciples follow his wise teachings. The big breakfast "habit" is entirely artificial since we are not in need of nourishment immediately upon arising! The "no breakfast plan" has helped hundreds of chronic sufferers, for this practice at least gives the over-worked depurating organs less work to perform. Stop eating the foods you now have learned are the direct cause of your ailment, and you will soon find that "over-eating" and "wrong foods" will prove to be the major cause of your illness. Let "fresh fruits" cleanse impurities from your system and if this simple method is conceivably possible of restoring your health—isn't it worth trying?

Ailments traceable to wrong thinking can fortunately be readily removed,—in place of worry, anxiety or pessimism substitute positive kind thoughts. Fear is man's oldest enemy and continues to remain one of his worst foes! Banish fear thoughts from your mind for fear exaggerates abnormal conditions, eventually causing disease and unhappiness. "That which I feared has come upon me" has often proven to be the case! The seeker after health need not become a food crank or health extremist. Enjoy food, without fear or anxiety; all "good food" agrees with the person who cultivates constructive thoughts. Meals should be eaten in a thankful, cheerful frame of mind for "A merry heart doeth good like a medicine" especially at the table. A full life of contentment, health and happiness can be yours, for "As ye think, so shall ye be". Faith, love and hope, the three great human emotions are desperately needed in today's world,—we must have faith in ourselves, faith in mother nature's ability to heal, and to provide us with all things that conform to natural laws. FAITH must precede knowledge and our faith must be the highest and most complete faith of which we are capable, a strong vital faith in the Creator, in his guiding spirit,—for without this faith life itself would cease to exist.

(FINIS)

MEMORANDA

THE DEFINITE CURE OF

CHRONIC CONSTIPATION

ALSO

OVERCOMING CONSTIPATION NATURALLY

The Internal Uncleanliness of Man . . .

The Effect of Laxatives . . .

The Real Cause of Constipation . . .

Nourishing and Curing "Laxatives" . . .

Conclusion . . .

Printed in U.S.A.

Introduction

A little over twenty-two years ago the author of this booklet was declared "incurable" of Bright's Disease by orthodox medical physicians.

After four years of exacting study and dangerous experimenting on his own body — for many times he brought himself almost on the brink of death — he discovered the following truth: Disease is Nature's effort to rid the body of disease matters and eliminate waste from the system.

No matter how desperately ill you may become, Nature continually tries to save you. The goal of evolution is quality and not quantity and the weak and degenerate are wiped out when Nature's laws are violated.

Instinctively the voice of Nature comes to man in the same manner as it does to animals, "Don't eat! — rest — be quiet!" Fortunately for those of us who are acquainted with Professor Arnold Ehret's teachings, this warning of Nature has been made clear and need no longer be unheeded by man on the plea of ignorance.

Fasting and fruit-diet loosen and stir up the masses of bodily filth, and poisons are in consequence carried into the blood-stream with disastrous effects. A thorough knowledge of proper procedure is, therefore, absolutely necessary before anyone should attempt to undertake a cure. After having himself suffered for years through lack of this knowledge, Prof. Ehret has successfully solved the problem and has evolved a scientifically correct system, known as THE MUCUSLESS DIET HEALING SYSTEM.

The object of this booklet is to give a comprehensive statement of the deeper causes of constipation and how it can be DEFINITELY cured and not MERELY RELIEVED.

The Definite Cure of Chronic Constipation

By Prof. Arnold Ehret

The Internal Uncleanliness of Man

Chronic constipation is the worst and most common crime against life and mankind — a crime unconsciously committed, and one whose full enormity is not yet fully realized. It stands accused of being one of the principal causative factors of all physical and mental diseases. I know as a fact, from my practical experience with thousands of chronically diseased, that the life of man, and the extent of his mental and spiritual capabilities are largely influenced by the condition of the alimentary tract. It is certainly very important that the brain and nerves of man are supplied with pure blood, and are not dependent on blood, polluted with impurities, arising from an unclean alimentary canal. "Unclean" is too mild a word, when we are dealing with the worst kind of a filthy condition.

It is a fact that man, the product of the present "civilized" society of this much vaunted "advanced" twentieth century, is born in filth, because his mother, during pregnancy, is almost invariably suffering from constipation. And I say further, that while in this state, she usually eats two or three times as much as is necessary. This causes the so-called normal, more or less healthy man, to be somewhat encumbered from infancy. And to a much greater extent, is the constipated one — who is loaded with such a mass of internal filth, that it can only be called "indescribable." His alimentary tract, reaching up from the mouth of the anus to his throat, is filled with a morbid mucus — undigested, decayed and retained food-substances, all of which are in a state of fermentation and putrefaction. His intestines have never had a perfect cleansing during his entire life. At the conclusion of each discharge, the anus must be artificially cleansed, which shows that the internal walls of the intestines must also retain, after each passage, quantities of this same filth.

A physician of Berlin, whose life work was the performing of autopsies, stated that 60 per cent of all the corpses contained in the alimentary canal various foreign matter — worms and petrified feces — and he further stated that in nearly all cases the walls of the intestines and colon were lined with a crust of hardened feces, making it evident that these organs had degenerated to a state of utter inefficiency. Progressive American physicians are rapidly awakening to the fact that retained fecal matter is one of the chief causes of disease. Autopsies are constantly revealing indescribable filthy astounding conditions. One physician publishes the following::

"I have found a phototype of the cause of all diseases of the human body, the foundation of premature old age and death. Surprising as it may seem, out of two hundred and eighty-four cases of autopsy, held, but twenty-eight colons were found to be free from hardened feces and in a normal and healthy state. The others, as described above, were to a more or less extent incrusted with hardened, rotten, rejected food material. Many were distended to twice their natural size throughout their whole length with a small hole through the center and almost universally these last cases mentioned had regular bowel evacuations daily. Some of them contained large worms from four to six inches in length."

"My experience from day to day developed startling discoveries in the form of worms and nests of eggs, that we daily get from patients, accompanied by blood and pus. As I stood looking at the colon and reservoir of death, I expressed myself in wonder that any one can live a week, much less for years, with such a cesspool of death and contagion always with him. The absorption of the deadly poison back into the circulation cannot help but cause all the contagious diseases. The recent treatment of hemorrhage of the bowels in typhoid fever has shown it to be caused by maggots and worms eating into the sensitive membrane and tapping a vein or artery. In fact, my experience during the past ten years has proven, by the rapid recovery of all diseases after the colon was cleansed, that in the colon itself lies the basic cause of almost all human ailments."

That this revolting and indescribable condition arises from the almost universal ignorance of right selection of food, reveals why the "Mucusless Diet Healing System" is such an important discovery and development for the regeneration of mankind.

On the outside, the man of today is carefully groomed, perhaps unnecessarily and over carefully clean; while inside he is dirtier than the dirtiest animal — whose anus is as clean as its mouth, provided said animal has not been "domesticated" by "civilized" man.

Long ago Natural Therapy proved, that in every disease there is a constitutional encumbrance of foreign matter, a clogging-up of the system. That statement of fact is not sufficiently explicit. The encumbering matters, foreign to the body, and of no use to the system, consist of masses of accumulated feces, undigested food, morbid mucus, and retained superfluous water, all in a state of fermentation and decomposition. Truly, chronically constipated man constantly carries in his intestines a veritable cesspool, by which the blood stream is continually polluted and poisoned, a fact which only a skilled observer can at once detect by facial diagnosis. Official medical science and the inexpert layman do not suspect "constipation" when the individual consumes from three to five meals a day, while he is having one so-called, good bowel movement. Man imagines that his "comfortable fatted" body is a sign of health; at the same time he is as much in fear of a cold wind and "germs" as he is of the devil. When such a "well-fed" man who is usually constipated, takes a fast or is put on a "mucus-less diet" — as I have advised hundreds as their last resort — he will discharge masses of putrescent filth, fetid urine loaded with mucus, salt, uric acid, fat, drugs, albumen and pus, according to his disease.

The most surprising effect of these treatments is the immense quantity of the discharged feces and the fetid exhalation from both the mouth and skin. But the most important "discharge" is the elimination through the circulation into the urine. The urine of everybody will then show a sediment of mucus as soon as he fasts a little or reduces the quantity of his food, or makes a change toward natural, mucusless foods. Doctors call it "disease" and it is in fact a self-cleansing process of the body.

This self-elimination through the circulation is the body's most wonderful healing work of every disease. To control this process by food and food quantities is the only true, natural and most perfect therapeutic art of healing and is in no other "treatment" so successfully accomplished as in the *"Mucusless Diet Healing System."

This elimination — especially that of the sick man after a long period of misery, suffering and unsuccessful medical treatment — is man's "greatest event." He now realizes what he had never thought of — and what only a few physicians in the world have ever understood as I did, through thousands of cases — that mostly all civilized men are walking, living cesspools, due to chronic constipation.

All his former unsuccessful treatments now appear to him in a tragic-comical light. He now knows exactly where the source of his suffering is to be found, no matter what the name of the disease may be. He now understands that he was wrongly and ignorantly treated by the doctors who "suppressed the disease," without eliminating the filth, which was retained in his entire system, especially in his alimentary canal, since childhood, and which condition constituted the principal causative factor of the disease.

The Effect of Laxatives

I do not believe that either physicians nor laymen really know nor understand how and why the body performs the laxative effect of these different remedies. Official medical science knows very little about the "why" of the drugs. Their experience is based upon the experience only that each one has a "special effect."

All drug laxatives contain more or less poisons, that is, substances which would become dangerous if they were to enter the circulation in a concentrated form. The protective instinct of the body reacts instantly by a greater water supply into the stomach from the blood in order to dissolve and weaken the dangerous substance; the intestines are stimulated for increased and quickened activity, and so the "solution" is discharged, only taking parts of the feces along. This is the physiological explanation, and you can see that the effect is an abnormal stimulation of vitality in general, and of the intestinal nerves in particular. It is an open secret that all laxatives finally fail, because the constant overloaded intestines are being over-stimulated by the laxatives and thereby slowly paralyzed. To continually increase the laxatives year after year, instead of changing the diet, means SUICIDE — slow, but sure.

The Real and Deeper Cause of Constipation

Constipation itself is a disease, and a really "severe" one, at that, because in severe cases it burdens the system with a heavy load of filth, sometimes weighing as much as ten pounds or more. Disease as such is an abnormal, unnatural condition; even "orthodox" physicians agree on that. We should expire slowly and painlessly, when vitality is exhausted, had we not lived with disease and suffering. That cases of "natural death" are getting more infrequent nowadays is further proof of the depths we have sunken into in the "swamps of civilization."

Constipation — this most common disease — has not decreased or improved in spite of thousands of remedies for sale on the market, and in spite of so-called medical science; simply, because the "diet of civilization" is unnatural. The human intestines are not organized at all for this unnatural food to either digest it perfectly, or to expel the unused residue.

Very little is known about foods that are constipating, and those of the opposite kind. What I wrote and proved in my book, "Rational Fasting and Regeneration Diet," regarding the fundamental causative factors of all diseases, constitutes the deepest insight known into the nature of chronic constipation.

Don't you know that bookbinder's paste is made of fine white flour, rice or potatoes? That glue is made from flesh, gristle and bones? Don't you know how sticky these substances are? Don't you know that skimmed milk, buttermilk and cream are the best ingredients used to furnish sticky base for colors for painting? That the white of eggs will stick paper or cloths so perfectly that it resists dissolution in water? Every housewife and cook knows how oils and fats stick to the sides of a pan. At least 90 per cent of the "diet of civilization" contains these sticky foods and man stuffs himself daily with awful mixtures of them. Thus the digestive tract is not only clogged up through constipation, but literally glued together with sticky mucus and feces.

Herewith the "mystery" of chronic constipation is unveiled and the story told of the fundamental causative factor of all diseases. Disease is but internal uncleanliness — this simply states a true but woeful fact. Fruits, green leaf and starchless vegetables do not contain these pasty, gluey mucus substances and are natural foods — yet little credit has been given them by doctors or laymen. I will lift the veil and show why they fail to understand. Fruit acids and mineral rich vegetables saps — dissolves the pasty mucus encumbrances and fruit sugar causes and develops their fermentation and forms gases. This so greatly feared fermentation of the inside filth is another necessary stirring up "process" to prepare them for elimination. Acid and fermented starch and glue lose their sticky ability as soon as they ferment. If an average meat eater or a child fed mostly on starchy foods accidentally eats too freely of good, sweet fruits, a "revolution" in the alimentary canal, with diarrhea usually sets in (extreme cases are called dysentery (cholera), and fever is caused through the increased fermentation.

In severe cases, if a doctor stops the diarrhea, and the patient is fed, as is usually the procedure, the patient dies, because Nature was kept from accomplishing the cleansing process, and the partly dissolved poisons remain in the system, causing death.

The patient literally suffocates in his own mire of filth, accumulated during his life from wrong food material and over-eating. If he does not die, his case ordinarily becomes chronic, which means: Nature is continually trying to expel poisonous mucus and gases, in spite of all obstructions and counteracting remedies. The constipation merely aggravates the process. Instead of eating less and then only loosening foods, the chronic patient stuffs himself more and more with wrong foods, becomes fatter every day and even takes pleasure in his increased weight. In fact, this over-weight, called health by the misguided ones, is mostly accumulated feces — water — and various kinds of filth. In most cases of tuberculosis, these conditions are typical. Five to six meals a day and one bowel movement or even less — no wonder he takes on weight, looks "full of vigor" — but can never be cured.

Nourishing and Curing Laxatives

No advanced physician will deny the relation between any disease and constipation. But today people are far a-way from Nature and the truth, and they are kept more and more in darkness — when taken sick they do just the opposite of what they should do. The slightest indisposition, a little headache or cold, which is the result of insufficient bowel movement, is treated with more, and so-called better eating — inspite of a decreased appetite. This is the main reason why Influenza, the "Flu," became a fatal disease. Formerly "Flu" was as easy to cure as the harmless "Grippe" — a self-cleansing process of the body, mostly prevalent in springtime. Knowing nothing of "scientific medicine," germs, etc., the patient instinctively followed his lack of appetite, took a mild laxative and very rapidly recovered; usually he felt much better after than before the "healing" disease. Today, he is falsely taught that a germ is responsible — and not his dangerous unhygienic habits. He eats too much, which is against the law of Nature, instead of fasting, the way every ailing animal cures itself. But the amount of internal impurities and auto-toxins of man exceed those of any diseased animal. A long fast, therefore, would kill the majority of sick men; however, they would not die by starvation, but would become suffocated from their own poisonous filth. As an authority in fasting I know full well the reason why a fast is so feared by most people, and that it has been misapplied by laymen. It is a crime to advise a constipated patient to fast until his tongue is clean, before removing the "deposits of poisons" from his intestines. I could only succeed in curing very old, severe cases of chronic constipation by relatively long fasts. Man, in regard to health, is more degenerated than any kind of animal. He lost his reason, so to say, about matters of which he thinks the animal has none at all. Yet! his intelligence places him far above the animal and enables him to assist Nature to overcome obstructions and difficulties that could become dangerous. That is the philosophical sense of the Art of Natural Healing.

Therefore, if you want to cure chronic constipation perfectly and without any harm, you must change your diet, and instead of using foods which produce disease and constipation, eat really nourishing foods which loosen up, dissolve and cure. But people are ignorant regarding this truth just as they are about fasting, and they try to do things without previous experience or knowledge, and failure is usually the result. What I call "Mucusless Diet" consists of fresh, ripe fruits and starchless vegetables, for they are the ideal foods, and the fundamental remedies for all diseases. Of course, the application must be intelligently advised by a practitioner graduated from my school of the Mucusless Diet Healing System, or a personal knowledge can be received through the study of my book, the *"Mucusless Diet Healing System."

It is an "eating-your-way-to-health" treatment, and consequently the most reasonable method of curing, because wrong eating is the causative factor in all diseases.

These mucusless, nourishing and "laxative," that is, dissolving foods, form new blood; the best blood that has ever run through your veins — and at once start the so-called constitutional cure of the body. The circulation of the new blood, permeating every part of the system, dissolves and eliminates the morbid mucus, which is clogging up the entire human organism; it especially loosens the deep-seated impurities in the intestines and renovates the whole system. This, then is the great enlightening fact — why constipation not only can be perfectly cured, but why the "Mucusless Diet" cures when all other treatments have failed.

In severe cases of chronic constipation it is advisable in the beginning, to use as a help, a harmless laxative, to remove the solid obstructions of feces in the intestines; in other words, to eject the worst filth out of a clogged-up pipe system. Enemas consisting of clear, warm water are also a good help in the beginning.

Among numerous laxatives on the market those of vegetable origin are the least harmful. After many years of experience, I have prepared a "special mixture" of this kind. It has the advantage of removing the old, solid feces, obstructions and mucus, from the intestines, without causing the usual diarrhea and constipation as an after effect. It is to be used in the beginning only, as an aid, and will not have to be used continually. As soon as the intestines are cleansed from the retained masses of feces and other obstructions and the mucusless or mucus-lean diet is taken up, you will realize the truth of the previously stated facts. You will then perceive with both your eyes and with your nose that I have not exaggerated. And you will become convinced that the state of obstruction was not only localized in your intestines, but that all passages of your entire system were obstructed and constipated with mucus, from your head to your toes.

You will then experience the formerly unbelievable fact — that any kind of disease —even those considered incurable by all doctors — under my treatment soon begin to improve and are finally cured, if a cure is at all possible, simply because the source of poisoning of the system — the chronic constipation — is eliminated. Then the new blood, derived from natural foods, circulates "unpoisoned" through the entire system and dissolves and eliminates every local symptom, even in the most deep-seated cases; and it removes the impurities of the entire system, which were mainly supplied from the deposits of poisons and morbid mucus in the intestines, which condition is called Chronic Constipation.

Conclusion

"Life is a tragedy of nutrition" is a statement I made many years ago. Everyone knows we dig our graves with our teeth, but the saddest of all is the present-day superstition of 99 per cent of the people.— the most highly educated and the ignorant — the healthy as well as sick — the rich and the poor — that we must eat more concentrated food when weak or sick. Concentrated food, high protein and starchy foods are the most constipating which, as shown in this booklet, accumulate in the form of waste in the alimentary canal. The so-called "good stool" daily is in reality constipation and you may now see that constipation is the main source of every disease and that the average person suffering from constipation can only be healed perfectly by a diet, free from STICKY — GLUEY — PASTY properties and that is a MUCUSLESS DIET.

You may improve your elimination temporarily through laxative remedies — special physical exercise — vibration, massages and various other methods, but you cannot clean out the old obstructions from the alimentary canal and regenerate and cleanse the whole system as long as you eat the same mucus and toxic-forming foods which have caused and continue causing your constipation and all other ailments of the human body.

FINIS

Overcoming Constipation Naturally

By Fred S. Hirsch

Neither time nor money has been spared by the best talents known to the Medical profession in an attempt to unravel the mystery of constipation, its causes and cure. No drug has as yet been compounded capable of permanently overcoming intestinal stasis. The problem of constipation remains a "problem" after thousands of years!

Arnold Ehret in his book "Mucusless Diet Healing System" describes it thusly: "Constipation results from a congestion of a capillary circulation brought about through excessive mucus and impurities (foreign waste matter) clogging up the blood stream and tissue system, to the extent that circulation is impeded causing inability to discharge the natural flow of fecal matter normally". In other words, loss of proper peristaltic movement of the intestines causes failure of the bowels to evacuate the unwanted waste fecal matter normally.

It would almost appear repetitive to further describe just what constipation is — or how in so many different ways it can harmfully affect the human body, but only through constant reiteration will full enlightenment bring the necessary knowledge of this most important subject. The various painful afflictions resulting from constipation have been given many "scientific names" descriptive of the actual organ or particular part of the body affected. Constipation is a blocking-up of the human "sewerage system" and makes of man a "walking cesspool"! Can you think of anything more repulsive than forced retention within the body of putrid, decaying, germ-laden "sewerage"? Would you willingly reside beside an open cesspool? Most certainly NOT! And yet this is exactly what the constipated individual is doing. We use perfumed soaps to counteract body odors and resort to a "mouth-wash" to "kill" bad breath. Just so long as the type of food you eat starts decaying and putrefying if allowed to remain impacted between the teeth, then "Brush your teeth after every meal" is a must. It seems unbelievable that we persist in eating these very foods in the unmistakably false belief that they are essential to life! What further proof is needed that they are the direct cause of our ailments!

Within this wonderful body of ours is contained a natural, miraculous ability to overcome intestinal sluggishness and the many other various ailments to which man is prey. All that is necessary on your part is to provide the proper kind of food Nature demands to restore normal bowel activity. The method of correction is extremely simple, but neglect through ignorance or otherwise, to heed Nature's warning will eventually result in a complete "breakdown". There can be no compromise; you have violated Nature's law and a plea of "innocent" is unacceptable; you must now pay the penalty. Either prompt removal of all "surplus garbage" or else! The bowels are overloaded, and this "blockage" cannot be tolerated. The necessary vitality needed to carry on, is lacking.

A complete cessation of the causes is the only possible hope. Stimulating bowel action through use of violent purgatives is equal to attempting to spur on an already exhausted horse to further effort! Only through complete cooperation can you hope for a "pardon". What a surprising "relief" results in your physical condition through following this rational health regime.

The One-ness of Disease

There is only one disease, although its manifestations are various, and there is but one cause, and that is retention of waste matters. Bias, prejudice and erratic conclusions have always stood in the way of progress!

Presumably you are in earnest and desire to attain virile, vital, normal, good health — otherwise you would not be reading this article. Good health requires dedication of purpose and unwavering observance of all Health rules. "Wishful thinking" must be replaced with "Positive thinking"; half-way measures bring only half-way results. The power to heal is invested in the individual. We must therefore do our own curing! Is gluttony your supreme source of pleasure in life, and if so, are you willing to exchange it for other more worth-while enjoyments? Your acquired "taste-buds" will soon be replaced with natural desires and you will soon find yourself enjoying pleasure in eating as formerly. Social activities might change but new friends will be found to take the place of those who might misunderstand. Your desire to remain young, energetic and vivaciously healthy must prevail. When this takes place vital forces are restored to a normal balance and mental and physical alertness returns. Every mouthful of Natural food is delicious to the taste, and life takes on an entirely new meaning of joyful activity.

Physical Exercises are necessary

Strengthening your flaccid abdominal muscles is most important since proper bowel function requires strong abdominal muscular ability. Use of the "slanting board" is particularly helpful in building abdominal muscular strength without overtaxing your strength. Lie flat on your back and with hands clasped behind the head try and bring the body to a sitting position. You may at first find it necessary to have your legs and feet held down until the abdominal muscles become stronger. Walking is one of the very best exercises and a daily walk of not less than fifteen minutes should become a MUST, for walking opens up new avenues of blood circulation in dormant areas. You can easily combine breathing exercises with walking. Inhale sharply through the nose on four counts — then hold the breath four counts; now exhale completely for four counts, and again hold the breath four counts — then start all over again. Use pure sparkling water if available — otherwise distilled water with the addition of a few drops of fresh lemon juice to replace the minerals lost by distillation, you may drink as much as you desire between meals — but no liquids with meals. We must learn how to restore lost health in order to retain good health indefinitely.

White Blood-Corpuscle and Anemic Paleness

Man today is pathologically sick. The anemic paleness and pallid white skin are visual indications that all is not well! Health authorities agree that serious recognition must be given the matter of complete and thorough bowel elimination. Ehret states in his book the "Mucusless Diet

Healing System" — "Over-eating of starchy foods such as wheat and grain products, breads, cakes, pastries, and pies and the dairy products: butter, cheese, eggs, and pasteurized milk, (acid forming foods) tend to produce an excess of white blood corpuscles, mucus and similar waste encumbrances, all of which, directly and indirectly contribute to chronic constipation. To restore a ruddy natural skin color with its vibrant healthy glow; the "red corpuscles" must predominate."

Keep the colon clean.

How often have you delayed answering Nature's first call because you were "too busy", or the time was "inopportune", and many other reasons? "House-broke" pets become constipated from this same "delaying habit". Don't fail to answer Nature's call immediately upon the very first warning! Retention or delay for too long a period can result in reabsorption of the semi-liquid poisonous wastes in the intestines, directly into the circulation through the blood steam; the remaining feces becomes dry, elimination is more difficult and an impaction of the bowels results. The simple-headache, nervous tensions, muscular aches and pains, dizziness, lack of vitality and many of the common types of ailments, are directly traceable to constipation. Cellular degeneration causing serious ailments eventually follow, and unless we can re-establish healthy natural bowel movements through a thorough cleansing, disease becomes rampant. Here in a nutshell, lies the secret of disease.

With a clogged bowel system, illness is bound to be present. Despite the repeated medical assurance that "aspirin type" remedies are harmless, we are bluntly informed by the manufacturer that "relief" is "temporary" at best. Yes, indeed, it will require a lot of COURAGE, PATIENCE, PERSEVERANCE AND FAITH on your part — before the elusive Fountain of Youth is attained.

Maintain a Normal Bowel Functioning

Prof. Arnold Ehret in his "Mucusless Diet Healing System" claimed CONSTIPATION to be the primary cause of 99.9% of all human ills, including the so-called "incurable diseases" — ie: Cancer, Tuberculosis, Diabetes, Arthritis, Tumors, and many others. In fact, practically every ailment to which the human body is prey! Dr. J. H. Kellogg of Battle Creek Sanitarium shares this opinion for he stated: "ALL CANCER PATIENTS ARE VICTIMS OF CHRONIC CONSTIPATION!"

We herewith submit a "suggestion" — primarily intended for our male readers only, since women have followed this practice for thousands of years! The "suggestion" has proven to be exceptionally effective in aiding and correcting normal bowel functioning! Could it be that this is the answer to the age-old question, "why do women enjoy greater longevity than men, normally outliving their male companions by many years?"

It seems that both men and women find ready excuses for post-poning "Nature's call", failing to recognize the seriousness of the occasion! Please — for your health's sake, and beginning with RIGHT NOW! — promise yourself never to delay answering "Nature's call" IMMEDIATELY! It can prove to be tremendously important to your future good health and well being! To post-pone this important function is a direct cause of resulting constipation which eventually becomes "chronic". Strange, isn't it, that when hunger "calls" we readily find time to stop and eat!

The advice offered to our "male" readers is extremely simple and easy to follow! Instead of your continuing the present "time-saving" custom of "standing" upright while urinating we recommend "sitting" on the toilet bowl — in a squatting position and at the same time concentrating on having a bowel movement! This may mean a few minutes extra time — but it will surely prove time well spent in improving your health! Patience is required and possibly ten or more minutes may be necessary during the "habit-forming" period. It won't be long tho, — in fact, one or two weeks should find you happily experiencing "normal" bowel movements! We are all "creatures of habit" and this "good-habit" is surely definitely worth cultivating! For nothing can be of greater importance to all of us than GOOD HEALTH! "When you have your health you have everything!"

These suggestions are equally important for women who consider themselves too busy to spare the extra few minutes required. Yet, they docilely spend weeks or months recovering from a costly surgical operation. Decide RIGHT NOW to follow these simple suggestions — you won't regret it! Start TODAY — not TOMORROW, and make it a daily MUST, every day, for the remainder of your life! Remember — "Mother Nature" accepts NO EXCUSES! She desires ALL of her beloved "children" to be healthy. Are you aware that we normally should experience a bowel movement within not more than three hours after each meal! THIS COULD BE THE SECRET OF GOOD HEALTH!

The ancient Greeks made a practice of "sleeping off" all types of illness. Their hospitals were known as "Temples of sleep" and the patient was kept sleeping during the entire convalescent period. Actually what took place was that the body was undergoing the "fasting cure" and the digestive organs received a much needed rest. Our hard working kidneys, liver, stomach, in fact the entire intestinal tract require this occasional rest just as do the involuntary muscles of the body. Under normal conditions Nature takes care of this "rest period" during a sound undisturbed sleep. Going without food for a few days provides a physiological rest required by our digestive organs. Here's an easy experiment well worth trying. Upon arising drink a full glass of hot water to which the juice of one-half fresh lemon has been added and honey may be added to taste. For your noon meal the next three or four days eat only an apple with dried figs. Nothing else! The evening meal can consist of a green leaf salad, grated carrots and sliced celery. Such a series of short fasts of 2 or 3 days each, if followed over a period of two or three months, will prove most beneficial. Your sleep will be restful, you will awaken in the morning with zest; more vitality will be noted and your mental attitude toward the rest of the world might even improve! Eliminating "waste materials" is just as essential as sufficient food intake.

The Habit of Over-Eating

Overcoming a life long habit of "over-eating" is a difficult problem for the habitually constipated; "habit" is the motivating desire to eat rather than "normal hunger". The average "good eater" often comsumes as much as five times more food than necessary. Valuable energy is needlessly wasted digesting the surplus food which remains in the intestines in an undigested mass of decaying, decomposing "garbage". Nature's method of saving the individual's life from self-poisoning is to "store" this surplus waste in the tissue system awaiting more opportune time to dispose of same! These poisonous wastes are re-absorbed over and over again, polluting the blood stream. The source of supply of these disease-breeding wastes must be stopped. Every effort to remedy the condition must be initiated, aiding nature to cleanse the tissues and help bring about a normal healthy condition of regularity.

The use of chemical fertilizers and poisonous sprays have come into popularity because of their ability to increase crop yield. But sad to say — it has been proven that fruits and vegetables grown in chemically treated soil lack the proper vital mineral contents and they can also create an additional health hazard. Be as selective as possible when buying your vegetables at "super-marts" and when possible select those grown in organically treated soils. Many modern Health food stores now supply organically grown fruits and vegetables that meet these requirements.

Who Are the Constipated?

"Constipation is one of the most frequent conditions that the physician is called upon to treat, yet there is probably no other common disorder which occurs so often and is so badly managed", observed Dr. H. L. Cockus, M.D. in "Gastro-enterology" Vol. 11. Dr. Jerome Marks, M.D. writes in "Dietetics for the Clinician". "Constipation exists when an individual does not spontaneously evacuate the bowel at least once in twenty-four hours". This condition also called "Intestinal sluggishness" is the result of wrong living according to Dr. Robert G. Jackson, M.D. and we find in his book, "How to be always well" ie: "The bacteria of putrefaction multiply with numerous rapidity. They not only produce poisons that pass into the blood and burden the organs of elimination, but they locally irritate and could set up an inflammatory state in the lining of the bowel, known to the physician as colitis. Constipation may seem a simple thing, but its proper treatment is a matter of great importance to the well-being of the individual. Ultimate success requires close cooperation.

A gradual process of elimination depending entirely on the individual's physical condition is the proper procedure. Avoid trying to "rush" nature for it may become dangerous to stir-up the "poisonous wastes" too rapidly!

Survival of our Present Civilization.

We are not attempting to predict the end of civilization in claiming that if man is to survive — he must soon make a decision between returning to natural foods or continuing on today's accepted diet of demineralized and devitalized "foodless — foods"; with its certainty of sickness, painful ailments and a shortened life. All you need do is read the labels on any food package! The manufacturer adds certain preservatives to make his food-product a good "shelf-item"; ie: one with "long-keeping" qualities. Artificial coloring and artificial sweetener, makes the item more appetizing and the chemical additives are used for various purposes many of which are trade secrets known only to the manufacturer. Through a recent discovery a chemical spray has been perfected making it possible to keep vegetables, such as lettuce and other greens, as crisp and fresh for weeks — as when first harvested! The time is rapidly approaching, if our present civilization is to survive we must take action. We owe it to the unborn generation who will follow us! The poisonous chemicals used for "crop-dusting" and for spraying trees have succeeded in not only destroying the unfriendly insects but friendly ones as well! Our "good earth" contains many friendly earthworms and friendly bacteria, intended by Nature to fertilize and purify the soil, and they have become innocent victims of chemical poisoning! We are rapidly reaching the point where the soil can no longer supply the fruits and vegetables with the necessary minerals and vitamins required for our very existence! How much longer can life continue! Or perhaps, a better question would be — "How much longer will we allow this to continue?"

Many books on this subject have been written sounding their note of warning, and are readily available at any public library, but they go practically unheeded. It is too much to hope that sooner or later through increased experience our health authorities will accept this knowledge which is the only salvation for abundant healthful life.

Physical Suffering and Mental Unrest

More illness, nervous breakdowns and suffering from mental unrest has been caused through eating wrong foods than through any other source. It is fairly safe to say that the average person eats what he likes, when he likes, and as much as he likes without giving too much consideration to what the end results might be. So in searching for the probable cause of physical or mental breakdown, even in individuals who have lived more or less faultless lives "dietetically speaking"; we still find food to be the chief offender! It is of course essential that the individual recognize this fact and is self convinced; and willingly corrects his or her dietetic short-comings. While stressing the importance of food, we must not overlook other important factors such as the need of a happy mental attitude, nor sufficient sleep, nor healthy working habits. Sickness is much less likely to obtain a foothold when all of these facts are given their due consideration. Modern food preservatives and chemical additives were unknown when Grandma was a child and "gout" was a sign of wealth! It is unreasonable to assume that we prepare our meals of today just as mankind has existed on for thousands of years past! The Bible mentions the longevity of biblical characters. The present day art of food preparation is a recent discovery. Our forefathers foods were much simpler. With the coming of more densely populated towns, disease became rampant and they learned the "hard way" the lesson that "Cleanliness is next to Godliness". After the European and middle-east plagues that threatened to destroy all mankind, the very streets were scrubbed immaculately clean. Modern sanitation, filtered water, sanitary plumbing and public sewerage systems are presently a must in Western civilization, -- but we still fail to recognize the essential necessity of "internal cleanliness" for man himself, and the average individual carries around as much as ten pounds of uneliminated fecal matter in his body, falsely considering this extra poundage as being "healthy." Our Government Food & Drug authorities are graduates of the same colleges as the Scientists in the employ of the large commercial chemical concerns who through Research and Development in their respective laboratories concoct the chemical food additives. The Government maintains at considerable public expense large testing laboratories of their own, and while admittedly acknowledging that artificial coloring, chemically produced sweetening and similar food additives are known to be harmful in large dosage, and have been proven to produce many ailments, they are permissible — "acceptable" because only small portions are used in the food product and are therefore supposedly harmless.

We have more than sufficient and ample proof of the constipating effects of man-made "foodless-foods" yet hardly a day goes by but what some highly-ranked Scientist issues a startling announcement of having perfected a "patented" chemical concoction capable of supplying the required food concentrate sufficient to feed the entire present population of the world at practically no cost what-so-ever! While possibly on the same date, another equally well known Scientist warns that over 50% of the "under-privileged" in the United States are dying from "mal-nutrition"! The actual truth is the individual can no longer find proper nourishment in the foods they must now accept! Urging the discontinuance of poisonous sprays and chemical fertilizers is in the interest of food preservation! Try and imagine if you can the tremendous quantity of poisonous pollutants, — millions of tons of poison-dusts released daily by planes, automobiles, motor trucks, oil refineries, steel mills and factories belching forth poisonous waste gases and other poisons into the air we are forced to breathe! The health of every individual, man, woman and child is threatened. Every living creature, both on land and sea — yes every living plant; all are faced with eventual extinction, unless this most serious situation is corrected — and soon! Scientists report that an analysis of the purest snow known to man — taken at the extreme point of the South Pole contain traces of "atomic fall-out". Contamination of our Water and Air must not be tolerated at any cost! What percentage of the causes of constipation can be blamed on the chlorine and other chemicals now being added to the water supplies of our large metropolitan areas? And the Dental profession has joined the ranks favoring compulsory "fluoridation" of our drinking water on the basis of "fewer cavities" for the children! These chemicals are so destructive that they require "special containers" since chlorine can eat through a steel tank!

Mental Unrest

Constipation when caused through "over-eating" and improper food preparation is a prime contributor to the condition known as "mental unrest" and "nervous break-downs." Our Health authorities are aware of these facts and recognize that the human nervous system is poisoned by impurities from the waste products of constipation which enter the blood stream. Nature has provided many "safety devices" to insure that only the "purest" blood feeds the brain cells — but often Nature is unable to cope with the situation. Impurities in the blood supply to the brain, makes normal functioning of that most important organ, inefficient and befuddled. Prof. Ehret in his writings tells of many mental cases that came under his observation. Most of them responded favorably to fasting and proper diet! The "mental patient" in a majority of cases, has eaten foods especially rich in "protein" for many years previous to his "break-down." With the total discontinuance of protein foods such as meat, eggs, milk and cheese excellent results were obtained! Even some mental cases caused through physical injuries or sudden shock -- uncontrollable grief or severe fright; have been known to respond to a fruitarian and starch-free diet.

Medical Examinations

The value of medical examinations is not to be underestimated — but in a majority of cases, results and not cause is given most consideration by the examining physician. Nature has provided a self-diagnosis which Ehret named the "Magic Mirror." Expensive laboratory equipment is unnecessary to safely diagnose your latent disease.

—21—

The coated tongue, foul breath, clouded urine, putrid fecal matter, puffiness under the eyes, excessive release of phlegm (mucus) through the nose and expectoration; swollen ankles, offensive odors from both under arm and feet, inflamed eyes, — to mention but a few, are visible signs that herald in advance your failing physical condition. Perhaps you are one of the thousands of well-meaning individuals, who have dutifully undergone a series of physical tests, spent your good time and money for a "complete physical," and upon receiving the Doctor's report and being told that a corrective diet was essentially necessary; you "attempted" — although rather feebly, to do your part and follow the Doctor's good advice; — but through lack of "will power" "faulty" eating habits were resumed and you were soon back; "enjoying poor health." Very often, unfortunately, full realization comes too late! Hopefully you still have time, for "where there is life there is hope." But Nature must be given the opportunity and **you must cooperate!**

Longevity Obtainable

Man has undoubtedly shortened his normal span of life through excessive food intake and improper living habits. Modern sanitation corrected the past scourges of pestilences — Typhoid, Cholera, Bubonic plague, Yellow fever and Scarlet fever. Hundreds of thousands of lives were lost and entire cities wiped out yet man permits the contamination of his precious life-giving "blood stream" to continue unheeded! Medical practitioners now accept the possibility of man's life-expectancy increasing to as much as 200 years! While their claims are based primarily on the efficacy of modern surgery; ie: transplantation of vital organs, the willingness on their part to admit that the human machine is capable of continuing for this added length of time is quite a concession. Drugless practitioners on the other hand based longevity through a return to simplicity in our eating habits — especially the avoidance of **overeating.** All doctors agree that the majority over-eat as much as five times more food than the body requires. Based on this presumption; we use five times more "vitality" than we normally should, in disposing of food surplus. The Hunza people are a living example of what "simple" natural living will do for longevity! Women who have reached the age of 150 years give birth to children sired by husbands the same age and even older!

One suggested method of reducing food consumption is to follow a non-breakfast plan. We have health advocates recommending the first meal at 10:00 a.m. and the next at 4:30 or 5:00 p.m. Prof. Ehret, — a 'two-meal per day' advocate, suggested the first meal be noon-day and the evening meal at six p.m. Here is the plan I have been following over the past fifty years: Upon arising, a full glass of hot water to which the juice of half a lemon and pure honey to taste has been added. This helps cleanse the alimentary canal. Many ardent health disciples follow a "one-meal-a-day plan" eaten at about 4:30 p.m.; it practically means a daily fast! No solid foods are taken, although pure water or fruit juices are permissible. Whatever plan you follow, you will notice that the reduction in quantity of food-intake will bring about a gradual improvement in your health and constipation disappears! The sufferer from chronic constipation must seek **permanent** relief through his choice of foods from the vegetable kingdom, ie: fruits and green leaf starchless vegetables, since he has no other alternative! All vegetables are rich in valuable mineral content, ie: iron, calcium, sodium, magnesium, carbo-hydrates vitamins and especially, Vitamins — A, B & C. Fresh fruits and starchless vegetables are alkaline or "mucusless" whereas grains and cereals are "acid forming" and definitely "mucus-forming." Dairy products come under the classification of "acid-forming." When preparing edible "starchy" vegetables it is suggested that they be thoroughly baked, making them more easily digested. Cole-slaw, is prepared by slicing the cabbage finely, then adding lemon juice and a little olive oil (cabbage is often gas forming, and the lemon juice lessens this tendency). Add chopped celery to the mix. You will find it to be tasty and an excellent "cleanser". If desired a little salt may be added. Cooked spinach, beet tops and baked beets, can be added. This makes a most satisfying meal, which will also prove "laxative". You will find many similar Ehret recipes in his Mucusless Diet Lesson Course.

Basic Rules for a Disease Free Healthy Life

Constipation need no longer be a "mystery" for you have now been informed of all the measures necessary to overcome the most stubborn cases. Recognition of internal uncleanliness as disease producing should make you desirous of overcoming your constipation, and the few following rules are submitted for further consideration. Distress that frequently follows eating is unfortunately too well known! The pathological effects are not thoroughly understood at present by the great majority.

1) — TO LENGTHEN YOUR LIFE SHORTEN YOUR MEALS! Eat slowly and relish your food, for food must be appetizing and thoroughly masticated in order to digest properly. The first stage of digestion takes place in the mouth; hence the necessity of thorough mastication. To avoid over-eating it is a good rule to leave the table while still hungry! Avoid eating between meals!

2) — Avoid drinking any liquids with meals. This includes water, tea, milk, coffee, fruit juices and even soups. Wait at least fifteen minutes after drinking before you start eating solid foods. And wait at least the same length of time after eating solids before you drink liquids. Liquids interfere with digestion of your food when taken together.

3) — Avoid all harsh condiments and spices. This includes salt, pepper, mustard, catsup, vinegar, pickles, etc. They may stimulate jaded appetites but digestion is retarded.

4) — Avoid using butter, margarine and most cooking oils. Use pure olive oil where necessary to prevent sticking to baking dish. Starchy vegetables should be steamed or boiled until soft enough to insert fork easily, then baked for at least thirty minutes or until thoroughly dextrinized. You will find added flavor through baking and also the food becomes more easily digestible.

5) — Avoid all denatured and over-processed foods such as white flour and "ready to use" cake mixes. Prepared "TV" frozen-dinners should also be avoided. All nourishing content has been dissipated through the processor's use of food preservatives and chemical additives. A more nutritional meal would consist of a salad of fresh greens, cottage-cheese, tomatoes and one or two cooked vegetables. Or

better still a fruit salad with Yogurt or cottage-cheese. Dried figs, dates, apricots or raisins chewed together with a few nuts until thoroughly masticated, furnish the necessary protein the body requires. Avocadoes also have a high protein content and are rich in poly-unsaturated fat, but eat sparingly.

6) — Avoid constipating foods such as mashed potatoes with gravy, hot buns, cakes and pastries and cooked cereals of all kinds. Dairy products -- eggs, milk, cheese and butter, are constipating and form toxic waste poisons in the body and should be avoided.

7) — Avoid all frozen desserts such as ice-creams, sherbets, etc. Frozen desserts "shock" the digestive apparatus, and have a high acid content. They rob the system of valuable Vitality. The too liberal use of eggs and milk can cause putrefaction in the digestive track; normal functioning is impeded and poisons which should have been eliminated are retained.

8) — Since man is a "creature of habit" it is wise to take advantage of this fact. Make it a daily "habit" to visit the bathroom the very first thing in the morning or immediately after eating. Allow yourself ample time; concentrate on elimination taking place. Be willing to spend fifteen or twenty minutes if necessary — during the "experimental stage." It may require sometime before Nature accepts the suggestion! You may use bulb syringe — with luke warm, not hot water, when necessary, retaining the water at least ten minutes before rejecting. You will eventually be rewarded with permanent regularity, particularly if a corrective diet, proper physical exercises and deep breathing has been followed.

The Cleansing Diet

Constipation is a direct invitation to disease! Constipation causes a depletion in energy, and Prof. Ehret makes this clear in his book "Mucusless Diet Healing System" in Lesson 5. Ehret's explanation of how vital energy becomes lost through excessive "obstruction" is understandable. "Weight is disease" he states, "and you will lose weight at first through following a natural food diet especially through use of fruit juices recommended on the "cleansing diet" — but this 'weight' consisting of 'waste encumbrances' is the direct cause of your illness and misery." There are many excellent, moderate priced Juicing machines now available for making vegetable juices, at home. Apple or prune juice can be purchased at all Supermarkets. Fresh orange and grapefruit juice are easily made at home. Certain juices will be found more laxative than others. Prune juice is always available and is an excellent "laxative". Fresh coconut juice when mixed with fresh (not canned) carrot juice makes a delicious tasty drink with laxative qualities. Both fresh orange and grapefruit juice have definite "cleansing" qualities. Remaining on a fruit and vegetable juice diet for three to five days is not difficult, since there is no limitation to the quantity you may desire to drink. Drink as much pure water as you care to, and if distilled water is used by adding a few drops of fresh lemon juice to each glassful the lost minerals are replaced. This could be considered a Fast since no solid foods are eaten. When completing the experiment make sure that the first meal is a "laxative" one. Ehret recommended sauer-kraut eaten with fresh celery stalks. Canned sauer-kraut can be used by first draining off the liquid; add water and bring to a boil, then add one or two green pippin cooking apples, also a few dried prunes. Stew for at least an hour. The sauer-kraut may be eaten either hot or cold. You should experience a bowel movement within three or four hours after eating. An evacuation before retiring, is important since poisons loosened during the juice fast should be completely eliminated as soon as possible. May we suggest that you re-read Ehret's "Mucusless Diet" book wherein he tells what is taking place during the cleansing diet and just what to expect. Do not retire before experiencing a "bowel movement" — after breaking a fast — and an enema is recommended if necessary.

The average individual does not properly digest an ordinary "meat-meal" without putrefaction occurring. Needless to say this poisonous putrefaction occurring in the digestive tract may develop such ailments as; Brights disease, pernicious anemia, goiter, scurvy and even tuberculosis. There is little doubt that man's health would be greatly improved if meat is left off the diet.

The formation of our teeth and the length of our intestines prove that man is not Omnivorous, yet he follows the same omnivoral diet of the hog, and other omnivorous animals. Will-power to resist the perverted habits to which we have become accustomed, and the adoption of a frugivorous diet will bring about a recognizable regeneration in your physical and mental well being within a few short months!

Of course you know all about the harmful qualities of "cholesterol" and how our digestive organs find it impossible to properly dispose of any superfluous quantity. Cholesterol not only clogs the lining of the intestinal tract but can affect many of the vital organs of the body and Cholesterol undoubtedly plays a considerable part in causing constipation. Every housewife knows how grease and fats cling to the sidewalls of cooking utensils; especially pots and pans used in cooking meats. It is no easy matter to remove these fatty substances and a lot of scouring is required. Yet, without giving it serious thought; the innocent housewife feeds these harmful foods to her loved ones! Ample evidence exists proving the inability of the human digestive organs to digest or assimilate saturated fats and greases! The mistaken fallacy that meats are needed to supply necessary proteins to maintain a normal health balance, makes it almost "sacrilegious" to oppose this belief. However, many physicians bravely admit that dairy products (milk, butter, cheese and eggs), directly contribute to a large percentage of heart-ailments because of their high cholesterol content. Prof. Arnold Ehret, considered all fatty foods as being harmful and extremely constipating; clogging up the intestinal tract causing the entire system to become overloaded with their toxic waste. As we grow older the body's vital energy is depleted; through faulty diet, elimination is practically stopped; the digestive organs are immobilized and unable to function; toxic, putrefactive wastes are retained; nerve energy is dissipated; and we become seriously ill. Improved habits of living; eating only non-constipating foods capable of "cleansing" the digestive tract, ie: fresh fruits and starchless vegetables, become the proper procedure for regaining health! It is safe to say that 70% of the colons of the average person are impacted--some exceptionally so! "Grape sugar" is recognized as the energy producing food element by many Nutritionists and all fruits and starchless vegetables are rich in this life sustaining substance. The German chemist, Ragnar Berg in his book on "Food chemistry," classifies all vegetables and fruits as "alkaline" calling them "acid-binding" where-as grains and cereals; ie: Wheat, barley, oats, rice and corn as "acid-forming." In almost every instance, Chemist Berg's "acid-binding" foods are identical to those listed by Ehret as "Mucusless" and Berg's "acid-forming" foods correspond with Ehret's "Mucus forming" foods. Chemist Berg found such dairy foods as eggs, butter, cheese and 'pasteurized milk' to be "acid-forming" and constipating. Many Doctors recognize them as harmful because of their high "cholesterol" content. Prof. Ehret called them "mucus forming".

Positive Healing Forces

We can only hope to attain the blessings of "Positive Healing Forces" through following proven health rules. Natural foods, physical exercises, deep breathing—PLUS a cheerful mental attitude! We human beings, in common with all other animals possess the instinct of self-preservation. An inborn fear of losing our lives is strongly ingrained in our sub-conscious. It would seem unnecessary to tell what constipation is and what harm it does to the body; for no other ailment has been so thoroughly and consistently discussed. Constipation is the clogging up of the sewerage system of the body!

The need of Proteins

While we recognize proteins are essential in the human diet, we contend that Nature supplies sufficient proteins in natural fruits, starch-free vegetables and nuts to fulfill our needs. Many physicians acknowledge this fact but their voices are completely drowned out by those who still consider meats, fish and dairy products as a main source of protein. This conclusion may be traced to the fact that animal proteins leave very little residue. On the other side of the picture — we find that residue from fruits and vegetables is considerably more! This is just as nature would have it! The large bowel requires "bulk" before "mass action" or "evacuation" can take place. The residue from the decaying meat, fish and dairy products, being insufficient to produce a bowel action must first putrefy and is then absorbed by the circulation for elimination — while most of this poisonous waste remains in the blood

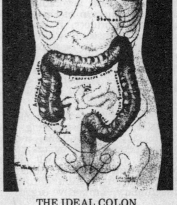

The Large Bowel or Colon illustrated above is classically in its anatomical position and scale. Considerable variation occurs in the normal colon depending on the type of individual.

THE IDEAL COLON

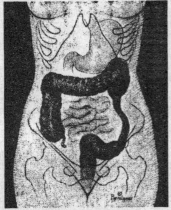

SPASTIC CONSTIPATION
Pinching down of the Descending Colon

SPASTIC CONSTIPATION

Spastic constipation presents a history of flatulence and griping pains in the lower abdomen. Physicians have looked for this type in patients with a highly nervous temperament. The bowel muscles are pinched down and contraction waves are too severe.

stream or is deposited in the tissues! The 'bulk-residue' from fruits and vegetables are properly evacuated since the main function of the large bowel is to rid the body of all waste products. If this process is turned over to the circulation; diseases which cause body-wasting and resulting weakness can be expected to occur! Physics and purgatives cause constant irritation and over-stimulation through constant use which ultimately may prove injurious. While "regularity" must be observed, to do so through means of a violent purgative is often worse than the disease itself!

Foul breath, coated tongue, mental depressions, loss of appetite, dull listless feeling, headaches, ringing in the ears, dizziness, skin-eruptions, indigestion, belching, gas-bloat often accompanied by cramp-like pains, ulcers and many kindred ailments are all the result of a long-standing constipation. Pimples, boils and other skin injuries are directly brought about through Nature's use of the skin as a secondary eliminative organ!

Man − a "scavenger"

Tracing man's history back thousands of years we find that he has long been a "scavenger" in his eating habits. He would voraciously stuff himself with the dead carcass of birds and animals that he had learned to slaughter even in his primitive stage. Not knowing where or when his next meal was coming from; he would gorge himself on the food available. His life in Paradise ended when he changed from his fruitarian existence to meat-eating! He has turned his intestinal tract into a "burial place" for putrefying,decaying animal foods. With the recent innovation of chemical "retardants" used to prevent "spoilation" in preserved foods, both bottled and canned; these chemical additives increase their "shelf-life". Even green vegetables are grown for acceptance in the market-place rather than their nutritional value! The search for greater financial profits supersedes consideration of food values! We pasteurize, homogenize, dehydrate, adulterate, emulsify and devitalize our food with cheap fillers, coal tar dyes, chemical bleaches, "U.S. certified" artificial coloring — (whatever that might mean) and even "formaldehyde" which everyone knows as an embalming fluid! Our leading manufacturers use "half truths" in their advertising, and very often even outright lies are told in advertising many of today's leading   food products. And we accept these food substitutes as "pure, wholesome food." Take time to read the label on the next loaf of bread you buy — or any of the bakery products for that matter! The Pure Food Laws require listing   of all artificial ingredients — yet the use of "artificial flavors", "propyl paraben" and other chemicals used to retard "spoilation" is legal. The effect these "retardants" have on delicate mucus membrane and the lining of our intestinal tract has not as yet been divulged — but you may be sure that they play an important part in the cause of constipation. Next time you are shopping — "pass up"the enticingly illustrated frozen "T.V." dinners and the patented "moist" cake recipes "so easy to prepare"! Stop cheating your body of the essential life giving foods. Every mouthful of fried, greasy food is a mouthful too much! Failure to pay proper attention to the desire for a bowel movement or to devote sufficient time to it, — leads to a retarded movement and later to constipation. Every individual living today is faced with the possibility of suffering either mental or physical break-down or both, through some expected, disabling, painful disease!   These almost certain results are directly attributable to present day living, — surely not an especially pleasing outlook! Increasing evidence has been found that habitual environmental distress, repressed anxiety, grief, envy, hate, fear, worry, and frustrations of all kinds cause constipation and often result in physical break-down, through organic changes.

Foodless Foods

A great majority of the people residing in the United States were raised on refined white flour products, refined and imitation sugars, artificial flavoring and coloring extracts, all of which are unnatural foods totally unacceptable by the human body. The discovery through illness in later life, —that only natural foods are intended for the human body seems to come as a distinct "shock" and total acceptance is not an easy matter. Adapting natural living methods will bring worthwhile results and this great boon of health and happiness is within your reach; grasp it firmly and hold tightly! Civilization, with all of its perverse habits has brought about the present decadence of mankind, proving conclusively the complete inability of the human body to adjust to an artificial, sophisticated manner of living. Only through living in harmony with Nature's teachings can these destructive disorders be corrected. Fresh fruits and vegetables remain generally undesirable to the average individual, thru hidden fear of possible harmful results! The teachings of Arnold Ehret have brought about an understanding of why and how the very foods actually "cleansing" the blood stream were wrongly condemned, tabooed and discontinued! Thru the teachings of this great benefactor of humanity, untold thousands now know the blessing of joyous "good health". Dr. J. H. Kellogg of Battle Creek fame wrote, — "Our health is made or unmade at the table! Your natural appetite will demand the foods your body requires, and it will be found that the easiest way is to consume food in its natural state. Whenever we eat "wrong-foods" — even though but once a month — our dormant diseased cells grasp the opportunity to resuscitate themselves and only through total abstinence from these "wrong foods" can you expect to completely free yourself from illness."

Arnold Ehret's Mucusless Diet System teaches that "constipation is a clogging-up of the entire human pipe-system. Nature wisely stores the undigested, toxic wastes "temporarily" in the tissues, awaiting an early opportunity to dispose of these poisons! Sickness is such an opportunity — "acute disease" is Nature's attempt to eliminate the stored-up "sewerage" and the "healing process" differs according to the physical condition of each individual". Most emphatically — we cannot afford to ignore constipation as a minor ailment! The very secret of Vitality lies in the ability of the body to eliminate these waste materials clogging the tissues and the intestinal tract. It is your duty to aid Nature's efforts through eating natural foods to keep yourself free from disease!

More Causes of Constipation

Eating a large breakfast of indigestible proteins, such as "hot cakes," waffles, French toast, oat-meal, bacon and eggs — washed down with a large cup of hot coffee — rushing to work immediately upon rising — often with insufficient sleep — makes it practically impossible for the digestive organs to function at all. And the final result is a deep-rooted constipated condition! Add to all this the combination of sedentary habits, plus a "one-sided" heavy starch — "bread, meat and mashed potato" diet!Constipation, being basic to every disease known to man-kind, from the simple cold to pneumonia — makes it difficult to understand how the average individual still believes in a "cure" merely through taking a "4-way pill"; an "anti-cold" tablet or some "patent" medicine.

We quote from a recent newspaper article:

"Millions of Americans falsely assume that there are easy ways to stay well and youthful looking, and resist the necessary arduous and disciplinary requirements of really caring for the complex, finely tuned, vulnerable body each of us inherits. Instead they turn, among other things, to diet fads, patent medicines, a countless variety of pills, and inadequate exercise. Our affluence has reduced physical exertion and increased "over-eating," excess drinking, smoking, late hours and drug consumption. A false sense of well-being leads many people to assume that illness cannot strike them, or that cures are to be taken for granted, laboring under the illusion that "miracles of medicine will keep them well"! End of quote. We thank you Doctor for you most excellent summation of the facts.

The simplest Meals are BEST!

Starting with today — instead of your customary meal of "meat, bread and mashed potatoes" try eating a crisp, fresh green leaf salad, using grated carrots and chopped celery, plus the addition of one or two cooked vegetables (such as peas, or string beans, squash or beets, etc.) with a few slices of fresh tomatoes added. If bread is used it should be thoroughly toasted and eaten dry. Avoid drinking liquids of any kind with meals. If your preference is for fresh tree-ripened fruit make the entire meal consist of crisp lettuce leaves and the fruits you desire. All fruits blend harmoniously. No starches ie: (bread or cakes) should be eaten with fruit salad. After a few days of this type of food you will be delighted to note that worth-while results are already being experienced! Unless you are actually hungry — DON'T eat!

Dr. Jonathan Formam, M.D., English physician writes: "If we were to use the knowledge regarding foods that is now available to us, sickness could be wiped out in one generation!"

You should by now be fully conversant with the life-giving foods meant for human consumption; foods that are best for you — fit to eat — foods that produce good health, strength and vitality! But we cannot stress too frequently the dangers of over-eating — of even the best foods. There is much more danger in eating too much — than of eating too little! AVOID OVER-EATING!

Retain Good Health Indefinitely

We have always maintained that the condition known as "constipation" is a direct invitation for disease! The individual is deliberately seeking illness — just so long as he permits constipation to exist. There is only one disease although it has various manifestations. There is only one cause — waste toxic matters retained in the system! During every moment of life, waste is being formed by the destruction of tissue, and this waste must be promptly removed to insure good health! You will find it necessary to call upon your Will Power and Determination to follow through and overcome Constipation — but you will find the reward well worth the effort.

Eating natural foods will bring improvement in both your physical and mental health. You may expect to experience slight abdominal pains occasionally and possible "gassy bloating" accompanied by belching. Should the pains become annoying try drinking a full glass of pure, warm or hot water. If the pains continue, discontinue all fresh fruits restricting your diet to cooked vegetables only, — until the pains have subsided, before returning to the fruit diet. The aggressive elimination of the fresh fruits stir up poisons, while cooked vegetables are much less "aggressive" in their cleansing ability.

"Whatsoever Nature expels is waste and foreign matter. When the body is over-loaded with encumbrances — plainly the result of decomposing, undigestible, retained foods — these morbid matters must be eliminated - or loss of health through auto-intoxication will inevitably result. — Prof. Arnold Ehret. When normal bowel functioning is insufficient Nature resorts to other methods of elimination — ie: boils, carbuncles, ulcers, or an abscess — to name but a few. All of which definitely signifies that the body is desperately striving to eliminate this unwanted surplus. The commonly accepted belief is that these foods must be replaced — and the sufferer is incorrectly advised to increase the daily intake rather than decrease! Recognition of the truth takes place when the patient is practically at death's point. This terrible "tragedy of errors" occurs until we finally arrive at a full realization that "Nature's laws cannot be ignored". We must no longer permit ourselves to remain unimpressed with Nature's healing abilities! Normal health depends upon correction of "our" misleading errors. There are, of course, many factors that can cause constipation. An abnormally slow movement of fecal matter through the large intestine is most always associated with a large amount of dry, hard feces, in the descending colon. This condition results through neglect or failure to respond immediately to the defecation urge; in fact, quite often with-held and not permitted to occur. The prolonged use of mineral oils has been known to bring about severe constipation, as do many of the commonly used constipation remedies. Both prescription as well as non-prescription drugs, including headache tablets, anti-histamines, aspirin, sleeping pills, muscle relaxants, opiates, narcotics and tranquilizers are recognized contributors and must be avoided! Practically everyone today is to a greater or lesser extent encumbered with latent, morbid matter which in itself represents a constipated condition, and the medical name given the illness merely identifies the particular part of the body or organ where the illness exists! Our blood stream supplies nourishment to every part of the body and only thru following Natures biological law, and eating proper foods as provided by Nature, can we insure our bodies a clean, vital blood stream. Natural health teachings are presumably techniques followed only by "food faddists" and "health cranks," and it is high time the unfortunate sick and ailing individuals exchange their "blind-faith" in the "surgeons scalpel" and dependency of medical drugs in the hope of overcoming their ailments — for the aid that Nature offers! The versatility and magnitude of natural healing has been conclusively proven over the years — even though medical science has as yet failed to arrive at a willingness to accept these basic facts.

In Conclusion

Our colon is the seat of all disease and therefore the preservation and restoration of health is solely dependent upon Internal Cleanliness! Life itself consists of a continual process of tearing down and building anew.

The average individual carries around as much as ten pounds of uneliminated feces. Continually carrying this mass of filth — day after day during his entire life, reabsorbing its poisons back into the circulation is surely a detriment to health. The engorged intestines, reeking with filth and putrefaction, poison the blood stream which feeds every vital organ. These poisons are steadily being reabsorbed into the circulation while in a semi-liquid state. A constant circulation takes place between the fluid content of the bowel causing every portion of this poisonous blood to pass several times during a twenty-four hour period, — into the alimentary canal.

The so-called "daily bowel movement" is no assurance that the individual is not the victim of costiveness, since the age-old, solid encrustations clinging to the intestinal wall permit passage of fecal matter through a small aperture of the intestines permitting daily bowel functioning to take place. An unnatural distension of the colon to several times its normal size results; and this impact colon is a veritable hot-bed for breeding disease germs and poisonous toxins. An exclusive diet of natural foods -- (fruits and starchless vegetables) purifies and cleanses the colon!

Health is an inestimable blessing; never fully appreciated until it has slipped from our grasp! Perfect health is the spice of life, and may those who enjoy this blessing retain it indefinitely! May those who have lost it regain it soon so that they may realize the joy of living! Nothing worthwhile comes easily!

Nature alone heals all ailments and only through complete acceptance of Nature's teachings can the survival of civilization be assured. FAITH, PERSEVERANCE, PERSISTENCE and WILL POWER contain the necessary ingredients to bring about GOOD health and the ability to OVERCOME CONSTIPATION NATURALLY.

"The journey of a thousand miles starts with but a single step!" (Chinese proverb) — We wish you "God speed" on your journey to better health!

FINIS

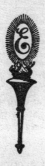

LIST OF OTHER PUBLICATIONS
By
PROF. ARNOLD EHRET

MUCUSLESS DIET HEALING SYSTEM— A complete workable Lesson Course for cleansing, rebuilding and maintaining a HEALTHY body. Explains fully in plain, simple, understandable language Prof. Arnold Ehret's methods for overcoming ailments through natural living.

PHYSICAL FITNESS THROUGH A SUPERIOR DIET— Also includes an article by Prof. Arnold, Ehret entitled A RELIGIOUS CONCEPT OF PHYSICAL, SPIRITUAL AND MENTAL DIETETICS wherein the author shows that a high degree of civilization can be developed through Physical Culture, Fasting, and Dietetics.

THUS SPEAKETH THE STOMACH also THE TRAGEDY OF NUTRITION— Revised and enlarged. A novel approach in which the author, Prof. Arnold Ehret, lets the stomach, the germinating center of all disease, tell the story of the tragedy of man's nutrition.

THE EHRET HEALTH CLUB

The Ehret Health Club was formed in the 1920's in response to the many requests from Ehretists around the world. The purpose of the club is to promote Prof. Arnold Ehret's teachings, and create a forum where people can get more information, and relate experiences, ideas, energies, suggestions, recipes, etc.

Let's work together to accomplish a task begun years ago by Prof. Ehret.

Let's strive to attain a healthier, calmer and more aware world.

For information, please write to:

Ehret Health Club
EHRET LITERATURE PUBLISHING CO., INC.
P.O Box 24
Dobbs Ferry, NY. 10522-0024